Hand Surgery in Asia and Europe

Editors

JIN BO TANG
GREY GIDDINS

HAND CLINICS

www.hand.theclinics.com

Consulting Editor
KEVIN C. CHUNG

August 2017 • Volume 33 • Number 3

ELSEVIER

1600 John F. Kennedy Boulevard • Suite 1800 • Philadelphia, Pennsylvania, 19103-2899

http://www.theclinics.com

HAND CLINICS Volume 33, Number 3
August 2017 ISSN 0749-0712, ISBN-13: 978-0-323-53233-4

Editor: Lauren Boyle
Developmental Editor: Kristen Helm

Hand Clinics (ISSN 0749-0712) is published quarterly by Elsevier Inc., 360 Park Avenue South, New York, NY 10010-1710. Months of publication are February, May, August, and November. Business and Editorial Offices: 1600 John F. Kennedy Blvd., Ste. 1800, Philadelphia, PA 19103-2899. Customer Service Office: 3251 Riverport Lane, Maryland Heights, MO 63043. Periodicals postage paid at New York, NY and at additional mailing offices. Subscription price is $398.00 per year (domestic individuals), $721.00 per year (domestic institutions), $100.00 per year (domestic students/residents), $454.00 per year (Canadian individuals), $839.00 per year (Canadian institutions), $541.00 per year (international individuals), $839.00 per year (international institutions), and $256.00 per year (international and Canadian students/residents). Foreign air speed delivery is included in all *Clinics* subscription prices. All prices are subject to change without notice. **POSTMASTER:** Send address changes to *Hand Clinics*, Elsevier Health Sciences Division, Subscription Customer Service, 3251 Riverport Lane, Maryland Heights, MO 63043. Customer Service (orders, claims, online, change of address): Elsevier Health Sciences Division, Subscription **Customer Service, 3251 Riverport Lane, Maryland Heights, MO 63043. Tel: 1-800-654-2452 (U.S. and Canada); 314-447-8871 (outside U.S. and Canada). Fax: 314-447-8029. E-mail: journalscustomerservice-usa@elsevier.com (for print support); journalsonlinesupport-usa@elsevier.com (for online support).**

Reprints. For copies of 100 or more of articles in this publication, please contact the Commercial Reprints Department, Elsevier Inc., 360 Park Avenue South, New York, New York 10010-1710. Tel.: 212-633-3874; Fax: 212-633-3820; E-mail: reprints@elsevier.com.

Hand Clinics is covered in *MEDLINE/PubMed (Index Medicus), Current Contents/Clinical Medicine, EMBASE/Excerpta Medica,* and *ISI/BIOMED.*

Contributors

CONSULTING EDITOR

KEVIN C. CHUNG, MD, MS
Chief of Hand Surgery, The University of Michigan Health System, Charles B.G. De Nancrede Professor of Plastic Surgery and Orthopaedic Surgery, Assistant Dean for Faculty Affairs, Associate Director of Global REACH, University of Michigan Medical School, Ann Arbor, Michigan

EDITORS

JIN BO TANG, MD
Professor and Chair, Department of Hand Surgery, Affiliated Hospital of Nantong University, Chair, The Hand Surgery Research Center, Nantong, Jiangsu, China; Editor-in-Chief, The Journal of Hand Surgery (European Volume), Edenham, United Kingdom

GREY GIDDINS, FRCS (Orth), EDHS
Consultant Orthopaedic and Hand Surgeon, The Hand to Elbow Clinic, Visiting Professor, University of Bath, Editor-in-Chief, The Journal of Hand Surgery (European Volume) (2012-2016), Bath, United Kingdom

AUTHORS

YUKIO ABE, MD, PhD
Director, Department of Orthopaedic Surgery, Saiseikai Shimonoseki General Hospital, Shimonoseki, Yamaguchi, Japan

GOO HYUN BAEK, MD, PhD
Professor and Chair, Department of Orthopedic Surgery, Seoul National University College of Medicine, Jongno-gu, Seoul, Korea

BRUNO BATTISTON, MD, PhD
Consultant, U.O.C Orthopaedics, Traumatology and Hand Surgery, U.O.D. Microsurgery, C.T.O. Hospital, Turin, Italy

REENA BHATT, MD
Visiting Attending Surgeon, Department of Hand and Foot Surgery, Shandong Provincial Hospital, Jinan, Shandong, China

MICHEL E.H. BOECKSTYNS, MD, PhD
Consultant, CFR Hospitals, Hellerup, Denmark

MAURIZIO CALCAGNI, PD, MD
Deputy Clinic Director, Plastic Surgery and Hand Surgery Division, University Hospital Zurich, Zurich, Switzerland

JING CHEN, MD
Lecturer and Attending Surgeon, Department of Hand Surgery, The Hand Surgery Research Center, Affiliated Hospital of Nantong University, Nantong, Jiangsu, China

KEVIN C. CHUNG, MD, MS
Chief of Hand Surgery, The University of Michigan Health System, Charles B.G. De Nancrede Professor of Plastic Surgery and Orthopaedic Surgery, Assistant Dean for Faculty Affairs, Associate Director of Global REACH, University of Michigan Medical School, Ann Arbor, Michigan

DAVIDE CICLAMINI, MD
U.O.C Orthopaedics, Traumatology and Hand
Surgery, U.O.D. Microsurgery, C.T.O. Hospital,
Turin, Italy

JOSEPH DIAS, MD, FRCS, MBBS
Professor of Hand and Orthopaedic Surgery,
University Hospitals of Leicester, Leicester,
United Kingdom

DAVID ELLIOT, MA, BM BCh, FRCS
Consultant, St Andrew's Centre for Plastic
Surgery and Burns, Broomfield Hospital,
Broomfield, United Kingdom

MARC GARCIA-ELIAS, MD, PhD
Consultant, Hand and Upper Limb Specialists,
Institut Kaplan, Department of Anatomy,
Facultat de Medicina, Universitat de
Barcelona, Barcelona, Spain

GREY GIDDINS, FRCS (Orth), EDHS
Consultant Orthopaedic and Hand Surgeon,
The Hand to Elbow Clinic, Visiting Professor,
University of Bath, Editor-in-Chief, The
Journal of Hand Surgery (European Volume)
(2012-2016), Bath, United Kingdom

THOMAS GIESEN, MD
Consultant, Plastic Surgery and Hand Surgery
Division, University Hospital Zurich, Zurich,
Switzerland

KE TONG GONG, MD
Professor and Chair, Department of Hand
Surgery, Tianjing Hospital, Tianjing, China

DANIEL B. HERREN, MD, MHA
Consultant, Hand Surgery Department,
Schulthess Klinik, Zurich, Switzerland

GUILLAUME HERZBERG, MD, PhD
Professor, Unit of Wrist Surgery, Edouard
Heriot Hospital, Lyon, France

JUNYA IMATANI, MD, PhD
Director, Department of Orthopaedic Surgery,
Okayama Saiseikai General Hospital,
Okayama, Okayama, Japan

**SHANJITHA KANTHARUBAN, MBBCh,
MRCS**
Registrar in Trauma and Orthopaedic Surgery,
University Hospitals of Leicester, Leicester,
United Kingdom

JIHYEUNG KIM, MD, PhD
Attending Surgeon, Department of Orthopedic
Surgery, Seoul National University College of
Medicine, Jongno-gu, Seoul, Korea

HISAO MORITOMO, MD, PhD
Professor of Orthopedic Surgery, Yukioka
Hospital Hand Center, Osaka Yukioka College
of Health Science, Osaka, Japan

HIROYUKI OHI, MD
Attending Surgeon, Hand and Microsurgery
Center, Seirei Hamamatsu General Hospital,
Shizuoka, Japan

SHOHEI OMOKAWA, MD, PhD
Professor, Department of Hand Surgery, Nara
Medical University, Kashihara, Nara, Japan

TADANOBU ONISHI, MD
Attending Surgeon, Department of
Orthopaedic Surgery, Nara Medical University,
Kashihara, Nara, Japan

SHIMPEI ONO, MD, PhD
Attending Surgeon, Department of Plastic,
Reconstructive and Aesthetic Surgery, Nippon
Medical School, Tokyo, Japan

ZHANG JUN PAN, MD
Attending Surgeon, Department of Surgery,
Yixing People's Hospital, Yixing, Jiangsu,
China

BERNARDINO PANERO, MD
Consultant, U.O.C Orthopaedics,
Traumatology and Hand Surgery, U.O.D.
Microsurgery, C.T.O. Hospital, Turin, Italy

JIN WOO PARK, MD
Attending Surgeon, Department of Orthopedic
Surgery, Seoul National University College of
Medicine, Jongno-gu, Seoul, Korea

INMA PUIG DE LA BELLACASA, MD
Hand and Upper Extremity Surgery, Mútua de
Terrassa Hospital Universitari, Terrassa, Spain;
Department of Anatomy, Facultat de Medicina,
Universitat de Barcelona, Barcelona, Spain

JUN QING, MD
Attending Surgeon, Department of Surgery,
Jiangyin People's Hospital, Jiangyin, Jiangsu,
China

CORINNE SCHOUTEN, MD
Consultant, Department of Plastic and
Reconstructive, Hand, and Aesthetic Surgery,
Catharina Hospital Eindhoven, Nijmegen,
The Netherlands

**SANDEEP J. SEBASTIN, MCh (Plastic
Surgery)**
Consultant, Department of Hand and
Reconstructive Microsurgery, National
University Health System, Singapore,
Singapore

DAISUKE SUZUKI, MD
Attending Orthopedic Surgeon, The Hand
Surgery Center, Nishi-Nara Central Hospital,
Nara, Nara, Japan

JIN BO TANG, MD
Professor and Chair, Department of Hand
Surgery, Affiliated Hospital of Nantong
University, Chair, The Hand Surgery
Research Center, Nantong, Jiangsu, China;
Editor-in-Chief, The Journal of Hand Surgery
(European Volume), Edenham, United
Kingdom

SHIAN CHAO TAY, MD
Consultant, Department of Hand Surgery,
Singapore General Hospital, Singapore,
Singapore

PAOLO TITOLO, MD
Consultant, U.O.C Orthopaedics,
Traumatology and Hand Surgery, U.O.D.
Microsurgery, C.T.O. Hospital, Turin, Italy

SHU GUO XING, MD
Attending Surgeon, Department of Hand
Surgery, The Hand Surgery Research Center,
Affiliated Hospital of Nantong University,
Nantong, Jiangsu, China

XIANG ZHOU, MD
Attending Surgeon, Department of Surgery,
Jiangyin People's Hospital, Jiangyin, Jiangsu,
China

LAI ZHU, MD
Chief of Hand Surgery, Hand Surgery, Qilu
Hospital of Shandong University, Jinan,
Shandong, China

Contents

The protocol for primary flexor tendon repair in zones 1 and 2 of the hand is changing. This article discusses recent changes. Immediate repair within 48 hours is performed whenever possible. A 6-strand core suture is performed using the M modification of Tang's technique. The pulleys are divided to allow free excursion of the repaired tendon within the tendon sheath. To avoid repaired structures within the sheath being too bulky, the authors generally repair only half of the flexor digitorum superficialis. In some cases, the flexor digitorum superficialis is excised completely. Rehabilitation remains based on controlled active motion.

Hand fractures (excluding small avulsion fractures and scaphoid fractures) almost always unite with bone. The role of the hand surgeon is not to achieve bone union but to achieve stability in an adequate position, often with some displacement, and maintenance of good soft tissue gliding. This article establishes that many fractures treated operatively do no better and often could not realistically do better than with good nonoperative treatment. Yet many are treated surgically to satisfy surgical egos, the desire to produce excellent radiographs, or just the mistaken belief that current surgical techniques can improve on nonoperative treatment.

There are increasing numbers of proximal interphalangeal (PIP) arthroplasties performed in Europe. Meanwhile, most surgeons prefer arthroplasty over arthrodesis. Silastic arthroplasties remain the most widely used implants. The main disadvantage of the Silastic implants is the limited stability they provide. Correction of pre-existing deformation is difficult. Soft tissue handling and postoperative scarring have an influence on the results of PIP arthroplasty. Different surgical approaches are possible. The most popular approach in Europe is dorsal. Different surface replacement implants are on the market in Europe. The main advantage of these implants is the lateral stability provided through their more anatomic form.

Scaphoid fractures account for 2% of all fractures. In Europe, the incidence is 12.4/100,000/y. This article focuses on the European perspective on understanding and management of these injuries. These fractures occur in young, active patients. The aim of treatment is union. Osteoarthritis is almost inevitable if the fracture does not unite. Cast immobilization is the treatment of choice in occult or stable fractures with 90% to 95% healing. Acute/primary surgery may be considered in some patients. The European literature stresses the importance of taking the patient's wishes into consideration after careful counseling about alternative treatment methods.

Recent laboratory research has disclosed that carpal ligaments exhibit different kinetic behaviors depending on the direction and point of application of the forces being applied to the wrist. The so-called helical antipronation ligaments are mostly active when the wrist is axially loaded, whereas the helical antisupination ligaments constrain supination torques to the distal row. This novel way of interpreting the function of the carpal ligaments may help in developing better strategies to treat carpal instabilities.

Current European Practice in Wrist Arthroplasty   521

Michel E.H. Boeckstyns and Guillaume Herzberg

The results of wrist arthroplasty for severely destroyed and painful wrists are generally good in pain reduction, increased grip strength, and upper limb function. The wrist range of motion is usually preserved but not improved. Implant survival seems better than it was with earlier implant designs; however, there are problems of carpal component loosening. Patient selection plays an important role, requiring experience, careful patient information, and discussing the pros and cons of arthroplasty and partial or total wrist arthrodesis.

Treatment of Intra-articular Distal Radius Fractures   529

Shohei Omokawa, Yukio Abe, Junya Imatani, Hisao Moritomo, Daisuke Suzuki, and Tadanobu Onishi

This review of current literature discusses the morphology of the volar aspect of the distal radius; the surgical procedure, arthroscopic findings, and clinical results of a plate presetting and arthroscopic reduction technique for acute intra-articular fractures; and a novel simulation guidance system for malunited intra-articular fractures. Classification of intra-articular distal radius fractures is also discussed, focusing on central depression fracture fragments, associated soft tissue injuries, and results for measuring scapholunate distances at different sites. Problems of the distal radioulnar joint are reviewed, in particular, functional outcomes of the authors' prospective cohort study on unstable intra-articular fractures involving the distal radioulnar joint.

Peripheral Nerve Defects: Overviews of Practice in Europe   545

Bruno Battiston, Paolo Titolo, Davide Ciclamini, and Bernardino Panero

Many surgical techniques are available for the repair of peripheral nerve defects. Autologous nerve grafts are the gold standard for most clinical conditions. In selected cases, alternative types of reconstructions are performed to fill the nerve gap. Non-nervous autologous tissue–based conduits or synthetic ones are alternatives to nerve autografts. Allografts represent another new field of interest. Decision making in the treatment of nerve defects is based on timing of referral, level of the injury, type of lesion, and size of any gap. This review focuses on current clinical practice, influenced by the numerous new experimental researches.

Mobilization of Joints of the Hand with Symphalangism   551

Goo Hyun Baek, Jihyeung Kim, and Jin Woo Park

This article classifies symphalangism of the hand into three grades and suggests surgical indications. Grade I and early grade II joints can be mobilized with early surgical intervention. Surgical results may vary but even a 20° gain in motion could be helpful for children and their parents. Postoperative passive range-of-motion exercises are very important in maintaining mobility of the joints. It is important that the parents understand exercise may cause some pain and they must be motivated to help their children during the rehabilitation period.

Jin Bo Tang, Grey Giddins, Shohei Omokawa, Michel E.H. Boeckstyns, Shian Chao Tay, and Thomas Giesen

Common hand problems are treated differently in different countries. This article attempts to bring together the views of surgeons from different countries on some of the most common hand problems that hand surgeons encounter in daily practice. In practice, the correct treatment of these problems may be the most important and influential to patients.

HAND CLINICS

HAND CLINICS

Preface

Evolution and Current Status of Hand Surgery Practice in Asia and Europe

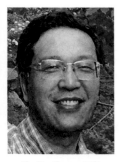
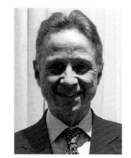

Jin Bo Tang, MD   Grey Giddins, FRCS (Orth), EDHS

Editors

Many hand problems were recognized first by European surgeons, and their management developed in Europe. Recently, the number of hand surgeons in Asia has increased substantially as has their worldwide influence. In an age of instant communication, multinational international meetings, and international journals, it would be easy to assume that the management of a common hand problem will be the same in countries of equivalent wealth. In fact, that is to ignore the myriad of different influences that affect how we practice. For example, for distally amputated finger, cosmetic concerns in East Asia encourage more replants; the financial pressures and volume of work in the National Health Service in the United Kingdom encourage a nonoperative approach. Different methods of funding in different countries will also bias their practice. It is interesting and enlightening to know and understand how others treat those we treat.

Over more than three decades, the previous 32 volumes of *Hand Clinics* have not designated an entire issue to hand surgery in Europe and Asia, although surgeons from the two regions have frequently authored articles in *Hand Clinics*. We felt that it would be worthwhile to cover the current status of aspects of hand surgery in two regions in a specific issue of *Hand Clinics*. This proposal was immediately welcomed by the editors at Elsevier and the consulting editor, Dr Kevin Chung.

Our invitations to the leading hand surgeons over the two regions were warmly received, and high-quality reviews from well-recognized and reputed centers have provided a thorough review and update on their practices. While the reviews are mainly relevant to their own practice or the current practice in their respective regions, they provide unique and novel insights. Readers will note how wide-awake surgery has become increasingly popular, how strong tendon repairs have safely improved the outcomes of tendon repair, how the function of carpal ligaments is appreciated from a different viewpoint, how conservative treatment should be an important, frequent, and efficient tool for hand fractures, how European colleagues treat difficult finger joint problems, and how Asian surgeons use vascularized flap transfers for immediate soft tissue reconstruction. Interesting and thought-provoking reviews can also be found on the topics of congenital hand disorders, peripheral nerve repair, scaphoid fractures, and wrist replacement.

In the final article of the issue, six senior hand surgeons from six countries were invited to offer their views, experience, and comments on a few common clinical problems. Reading this review is to experience a traveling fellowship; like conventional traveling fellowship, these views provide eye-opening experiences to challenge and enhance our knowledge. Through this article, the

Hand Clin 33 (2017) xiii–xiv
http://dx.doi.org/10.1016/j.hcl.2017.05.001
0749-0712/17/© 2017 Published by Elsevier Inc.

readers are led on a tour in these hand centers with senior hand surgeons explaining how some common hand problems are treated in their centers. Though there is common ground in their different approaches, there are also striking differences in the management between different centers and different countries. Besides inspiration from the different approaches, the contents should stimulate us to further explore that which we do not know, or do not know for sure.

In Asia and Europe there is a federation of societies for hand surgery in each of the two regions. The annual congress of the Federation for European Societies for Surgery of the Hand (FESSH) is a major event of hand surgery each year. This year's congress in Budapest was attended by 1780 participants from 68 countries. Most of the authors for this issue are active in two federations.

We are very grateful to authors of the articles in this issue for their time and contribution. While aiming to provide an update on current major topics in hand surgery, we could not cover every important topic. We hope the contents in this issue foster communication between colleagues across regions. It has been a privilege to edit this issue. We appreciate the editorial team of the publisher, especially Jennifer Flynn-Briggs and Kristen Helm, for their consistent and careful support and guidance during the production process.

Jin Bo Tang, MD
Department of Hand Surgery
Affiliated Hospital of Nantong University
20 West Temple Road
Nantong, Jiangsu, China

Grey Giddins, FRCS (Orth), EDHS
University of Bath
29a James Street West
Bath BA1 2BT, UK

E-mail addresses:
jinbotang@yahoo.com (J.B. Tang)
greygiddins@thehandclinic.co.uk (G. Giddins)

Performing Hand Surgery Under Local Anesthesia Without a Tourniquet in China

CrossMark

Jin Bo Tang, MD[a],*, Ke Tong Gong, MD[b], Lai Zhu, MD[c],
Zhang Jun Pan, MD[d], Shu Guo Xing, MD[a]

KEYWORDS

- Anesthesia • Tourniquet • Carpal tunnel release • Hand fractures • Tendon repairs
- Tumor resection • Cost and efficiency of hand surgery

KEY POINTS

- Performing surgeries in the hand or forearm under local anesthesia with epinephrine, that is, wide-awake surgery, is a recent development. This approach achieves excellent anesthetic and vaso-constrictive effects. It works very well for carpal tunnel releases and treatment of hand fractures.
- This setting allows intraoperative active motion to check the quality of repaired flexor tendons. As the tension can be judged through active hand movement this is even more appropriate for tendon transfer.
- The wide-awake approach is also used in benign soft tissue or bone tumor resection, cubital tunnel release, nerve repair, and wrist arthroscopy.
- Wide-awake approaches have been used by surgeons in a growing number of hospitals. Some surgeons routinely use it, and some hospitals have operating rooms designated specifically for this type of surgery.
- Experience in China suggests that wide-awake surgery is safe, economical, and patient-friendly, optimizing hospital resource allocation and increasing the efficiency of hand and upper extremity surgeries.

INTRODUCTION

In China, most operations in the upper extremity are usually performed with brachial plexus anesthesia. A tourniquet is applied to the upper arm to stop intraoperative bleeding, and most patients are awake during surgery. Wide-awake hand surgery proposed in recent years, specifically refers to surgery under local anesthetic with epinephrine administered by the surgeon. This achieves both anesthesia and vasoconstriction in the surgical field.[1–5]

In wide-awake hand surgery:

1. The patient is awake during surgery
2. No tourniquet is needed
3. No anesthesiologist is involved
4. The patient can move the digits, hand, and forearm actively any time during surgery, at the request of the surgeon.

This technique differs greatly from the traditional practice of simply keeping the patient awake while using a tourniquet. It has gained popularity quickly

[a] Department of Hand Surgery, The Hand Surgery Research Center, Affiliated Hospital of Nantong University, Nantong, Jiangsu, China; [b] Department of Hand Surgery, Tianjing Hospital, Tianjing, China; [c] Hand Surgery, Qilu Hospital of Shandong University, Jinan, Shandong, China; [d] Department of Surgery, Yixing People's Hospital, Yixing, Jiangsu, China
* Corresponding author. Department of Hand Surgery, The Hand Surgery Research Center, Affiliated Hospital of Nantong University, 20 West Temple Road, Nantong 226001, Jiangsu, China.
E-mail address: jinbotang@yahoo.com

Hand Clin 33 (2017) 415–424
http://dx.doi.org/10.1016/j.hcl.2017.04.013
0749-0712/17/© 2017 Elsevier Inc. All rights reserved.

Table 1
The procedures often performed in the wide-awake surgical setting and hospitals

Procedures	Nantong	Tianjing	Jishuitan (Beijing)	Yixing	Qilu (Jinan)
Carpal tunnel release	X	X	X	X	X
Fracture fixation	X	X	—	X	—
Tendon repairs	X	X	—	X	—
Tendon transfer	X	X	X	—	—
Nerve repair	X	X	—	X	—
Cubital tunnel release	X	—	—	—	—
Wrist arthroscopy	X	—	X	—	—
Benign tumor resection	X	—	—	—	X

in China, partly because Chinese patients and surgeons have been accustomed for decades to awake hand surgery.

The term wide-awake hand surgery does not make much sense in Chinese. Local anesthesia without a tourniquet is better terminology in Chinese. However, for simplicity and consistency with terminologies in the English-speaking world, in this article the authors use the terms wide-awake hand surgery or wide-awake setting, to indicate hand surgeries performed under local anesthesia without a tourniquet.

This article reviews common procedures that Chinese hand surgeons perform in the wide-awake setting and the impact of new approaches to hand surgery are discussed.

PROCEDURES PERFORMED IN THE WIDE-AWAKE SETTING

Procedures performed in the wide-awake setting in different hospitals in China are summarized in **Table 1**.

Carpal Tunnel Release and Fixation of Metacarpal or Phalangeal Fractures

Carpal tunnel release is a popular procedure in the wide-awake setting in China, because the surgical incision is usually small and procedures are very straightforward.[6–13] Hand surgeons in China believe that among all the operations performed wide-awake carpal tunnel release, and fixation of metacarpal and phalangeal fractures are the most worthwhile and straightforward.

Intraoperative hand motion is another benefit, but of secondary consideration in these cases. On completion of surgical release or internal fixation, the surgeon asks the patient to move their hand to confirm gliding and correct finger rotation.

Uncomplicated carpal tunnel release or phalangeal or metacarpal fractures seldom require surgical incisions longer than 2 cm,[14,15] which makes these surgeries perfectly suitable for local anesthesia (**Figs. 1** and **2**). If severe carpal tunnel compression or revision surgery requires an

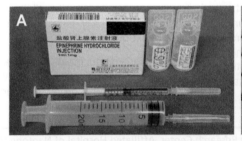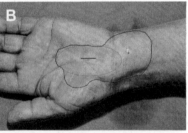

Fig. 1. Injection of local anesthesia around carpal tunnel. (*A*) Preparation of the injection mixture. The authors make the mixture freshly in China. Twenty mL of anesthetic mixture of 1% lidocaine with epinephrine (1:100,000) should be prepared and 10 to 15 mL of the mixture should be injected around the carpal tunnel area. (*B*) The area of injection. The area of infiltration (*red circle*) with 4 injections (1 proximal to the carpal crease, 2 at the area of the surgical incision in this patient, and 1 at the thenar area). For less severe cases, infiltration of a narrower area (*light blue shadow*) through only 2 injections made distal and proximal to the site of the surgical incision is usually sufficient for carpal tunnel release through a 2 cm incision. (*Courtesy of* [*A*] Shanghai Harvest Pharmaceutical Co., Ltd., Shanghai, China.)

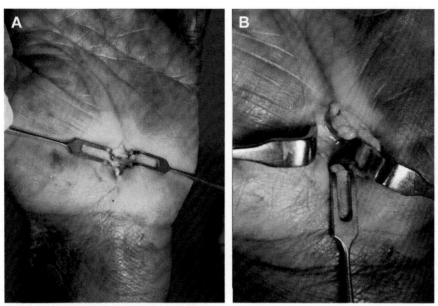

Fig. 2. (*A*) After making the skin incision. (*B*) Exposure of the carpal tunnel and transection of the carpal tunnel without bleeding noted in the surgical field.

extensive surgical incision, or there are bone defects in the metacarpals or phalanges, or multiple bones are involved, sedation of the patients or a brachial plexus block should be used. In addition, the authors emphasize that fracture wiring or screw fixation remain the easiest and most effective method for fixation of hand fractures and that plating should be avoided whenever possible. Plating a fracture in the hand is usually difficult in the wide-awake setting, but some surgeons (including authors KTG and SGX) plate the metacarpals using this approach (**Figs. 3** and **4**). They administer additional local anesthesia in the midpoint between the median and ulnar nerves in

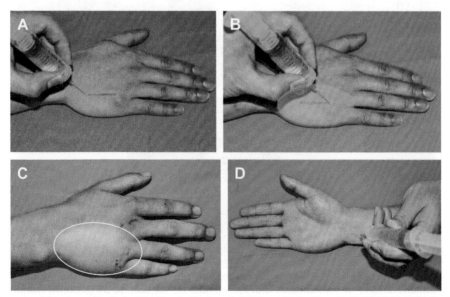

Fig. 3. The area of local anesthetic infiltration in the hand. (*A*) Dorsal injection site 1 (*light blue shadow*). (*B*) Dorsal injection site 2 (*light blue shadow*). (*C*) After dorsal infiltration (*yellow circle*). (*D*) Another injection (*light blue shadow*) can be added between the median and ulnar nerve in wrist level, with 10 to 15 mL of anesthetic mixture in each site.

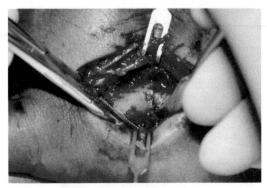

Fig. 4. Exposure for internal fixation of the metacarpal bones.

the wrist and anesthetics to the bone cavity and periosteum around the surgical site to improve anesthesia.

Flexor and Extensor Tendon Repairs

Primary flexor tendon repair can take an hour or longer to complete. The merit of the wide-awake setting for the tendon repair is

intraoperative active digital extension and flexion to check the quality of repair (**Figs. 5** and **6**).[16–23] In the conventional setting (ie, under sedation or brachial plexus block), repair quality can be confirmed through passive motion of the repaired fingers but active digital extension-flexion test should be more reliable. However, because the proximal tendon end sometimes retracts, requiring a separate proximal incision and extension of the operative field, many surgeons still repair tendons under conventional anesthesia. The authors believe the wide-awake approach will be used increasingly.[24–26]

Extensor tendon injuries, especially clean-cut wounds, are perfect for wide-awake surgery. Extensor tendons do not retract much and exposure is limited.

Tendon Transfers

This is among best indications for the wide-awake setting. The tension of tendons as they are sutured together can be judged correctly with the patient awake, with normal muscle tone and intraoperative hand motion, ensuring that the set tension is closer to ideal (**Figs. 7** and **8**).

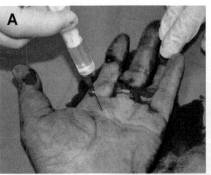
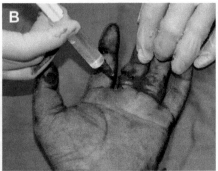
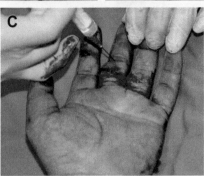

Fig. 5. The area of infiltration of local anesthetics for zone 2 flexor tendon repair. (*A*) The site of first injection, 10 mL of anesthetic mixture of 1% lidocaine with epinephrine (1: 100,000), at the proximal margin of zone 2. (*B*) The second injection of 10 mL of anesthetic mixture just proximal to the site of laceration, usually given 10 to 15 minutes after the first injection. (*C*) The third injection of 5 mL of anesthetic mixture distal to the site of laceration, immediately after the second injection. The fourth injection of 5 mL of anesthetic mixture can be given at the distal interphalangeal joint level if the laceration is rather extended.

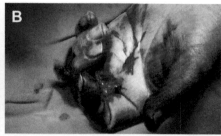

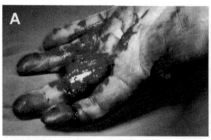

Fig. 6. The active digital extension-flexion test in the wide-awake setting. (*A*) Full extension. (*B*) Moving toward flexion. The test confirms the tendon does not gap during extension and the pulleys do not hinder tendon gliding during flexion.

Digital Nerve Repairs

An isolated cut digital nerve can be repaired in the wide-awake setting (**Fig. 9**), but if multiple nerves or other structures are cut, most surgeons prefer a conventional approach.

Nerve Repair in the Forearm and Cubital Tunnel Release

The decision to perform wide-awake surgery in nerve repair or cubital tunnel release of the forearm and elbow regions depends on the surgeon's preference, though the wide-awake approach in these 2 conditions is not as popular as for carpal tunnel release or tendon transfers. Surgeons can perform these procedures with local anesthesia, not all patients want to be wide-awake and there is always a concern among surgeons that local anesthesia might not be as effective as it is in the digits or the hand. However, some surgeons, including the authors, sometimes perform these procedures under local anesthesia. Before making a decision on a proper approach for the 2 procedures, the authors always consult patients and weigh their opinions and preferences heavily. Surgeons' proficiency

and preferences also play a strong role in choosing an approach. For those who often use the wide-awake approach, surgical release of the cubital tunnel is fast, easy, and reliable. Release is performed through a 3 cm mini-incision. With traction of the skin at the incision distally or proximally, the entire cubital tunnel can be released (**Figs. 10 and 11**). However, the wide-awake approach is unsuitable for obese patients or patients who are likely to need anterior transposition of the ulnar nerve or partial medial epicondylectomy.

Wrist Arthroscopy

Because the portals for inserting the wrist arthroscope are small,[27–35] local anesthesia suffices. Without general anesthesia or brachial plexus block, muscle and ligament tone is normal, and the hand can move actively, favoring assessment of the integrity and tension of wrist ligaments. Intra-articular bleeding is rarely a problem, even without a tourniquet.

Tumor Resection in the Hand and Forearm

This is a recent expansion of the wide-awake approach. Soft-tissue tumors in the hand and

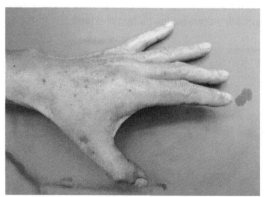

Fig. 7. Tendon transfer of index finger extensor for thumb extension. (*Courtesy of* K.T. Gong, MD, Tianjing, China.)

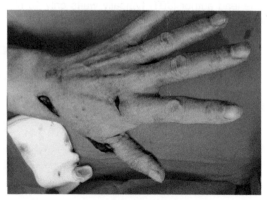

Fig. 8. Skin incisions and only minimal bleeding (in the gauze) during the entire procedure. (*Courtesy of* K.T. Gong, MD, Tianjing, China.)

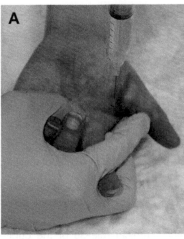
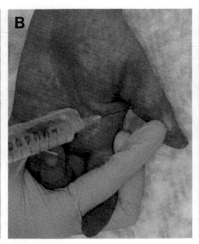
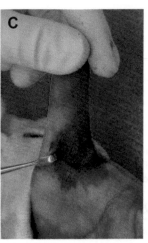

Fig. 9. (*A*) Site of local injection for exposure of the cut digital nerve. (*B*) Additional injections around the site of injury. (*C*) Exposure of the digital nerve.

forearm, and some benign bone tumors in the digits, can be excised through this approach. Many patients are satisfied with this approach.

Resection of ganglia or release of a trigger finger has traditionally been performed without a tourniquet or anesthesiologist in China. Therefore, this is not a major change in these procedures, but surgeons are more frequently adding epinephrine to local anesthesia.

VARIATIONS IN PRACTICE

Lalonde and colleagues have written extensively about the technical details of the wide-awake approach.[1–4] Surgeons across China differ in how they use this approach. Some variations are summarized in the next sections.

No Need to Wait for 20 to 30 Minutes to Begin Surgery in Most Patients

The lead author (JBT) typically waits only 15 minutes. At the time of skin incision, some bleeding

is noted but, as the surgeon reaches the deep tissues, bleeding decreases and the field is clean enough to allow for repair or reconstruction. Some surgeons in China start operating even sooner. Often, the time the authors wait depends on how soon the patients are brought into the operating room, which in turn depends on completion of the previous case in that room. The authors believe that there is no strict need to wait 20 to 30 minutes after injection of local anesthetics and epinephrine. It is, however, of no concern to start 40 to 50 minutes after injection of epinephrine if the previous operation lasted longer than expected. The effectiveness of vasoconstriction of epinephrine lasts 4 to 5 hours.

Supplementary Anesthesia to Deeper Tissues May be Needed During Some Procedures

In performing open reduction and internal fixation of the metacarpals or phalanges, or removing tumors from these bones, 10 to 20 mL of local anesthetic (usually lidocaine for its faster onset) are dropped

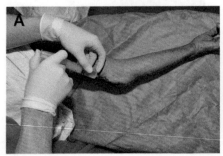
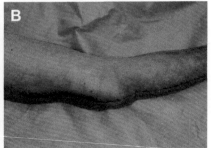

Fig. 10. Area of infiltration of local anesthetics for mini-incision cubital tunnel release with 20 to 30 mL of anesthetic mixture. (*A*) The first injection is made proximal to the area of surgery, followed by two injections at the middle and distal to the cubital tunnel. (*B*) After completion of injection. (*Courtesy of* S.G. Xing, MD, Nantong, Jiangsu, China.)

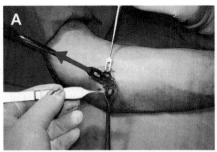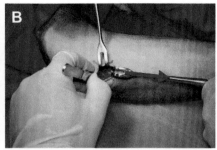

Fig. 11. After incision of 3 cm. (*A*) Proximal traction (*red arrow*) of the skin. (*B*) Distal traction (*red arrow*) of the skin to allow in situ decompression of the ulnar nerve. (*Courtesy of* S.G. Xing, MD, Nantong, Jiangsu, China.)

or infused into the periosteum and the bone cavity to reduce pain. The local anesthetic given before surgery is administered to the skin and subcutaneous tissue, which often does not reach the periosteum adequately. In addition, block of the digital nerves, or median and ulnar nerves, may be needed to ensure that patients remain pain-free.

Flap or Replantation May Not be a Contraindication for This Technique

Local anesthetics with epinephrine are not currently indicated in the dissection or anastomosis of blood vessels. Nevertheless, the vasoconstriction caused by epinephrine mainly affects the capillaries. With this approach, some surgeons perform replantation, as well as debridement and anastomosis, of large vessels in the hand although there are concerns about its use in flap surgery.

ADVANTAGES

Wide-awake hand surgery offers several advantages:

1. Lower costs to patients and hospitals
2. More efficient workflow in the operating room and, in particular, a huge saving of surgeons' time, because of quick turnaround time between cases
3. Reduced operating time through omission of the tourniquet and simpler surgical draping
4. Surgeons can advise patients about their postoperative care, including dressings, pain control, hand elevation, and range of motion exercises at the time of surgery.
5. No need for conventional postoperative recovery, speeding patient discharge and reducing hospital costs.

IMPACT ON DEPARTMENTAL SETTINGS

The impacts of this new approach are apparent in a few hospitals at the forefront of adopting this approach in China.

At Nantong University, a new operating room specifically for wide-awake hand surgery was created within an inpatient ward of the Department of Hand Surgery (**Fig. 12**) with capacity for 8 to 10 cases a day. The operating room nurses come from the wards, so surgeons have no restriction in deciding the time of surgery. Any surgery, whether outpatient or inpatient, can be performed whenever the room is empty. In addition, surgeons may choose to operate even in the evening. This operating room offers great flexibility to both surgeons and patients, saving huge amounts of patient time by avoiding scheduling and waiting. The doctors' offices are less than 1 minute walk away, and they can come quickly to operate. An operating room in the main hand surgery operating center is also used for wide-awake surgery (**Fig. 13**). In Nantong, more than 2000 patients have been operated on in such a setting over the past 6 years.

At Tianjing Hospital, wide-awake hand surgery is now performed every weekday in a major operating room. Hand surgeons have reached a consensus with the department of anesthesiology that local anesthesia is the main form of anesthesia for certain hand disorders, so that no anesthesiologist is needed in those cases. Currently, about

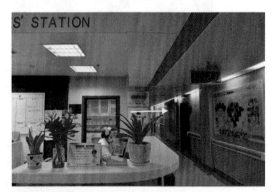

Fig. 12. The wide-awake surgical room (*white arrow*) inside the Department of Hand Surgery, Nantong University.

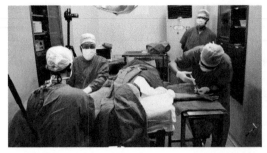

Fig. 13. The setting inside the wide-awake operating room in the main hand surgery operating center.

20% of hand operations are performed in this way, increasing the number of operative patients by 20% to 25%. Last year, surgeons in this hospital operated on roughly 500 patients with this approach.

In Nantong, the patient waiting area also contains a station for patients to select his or her favorite movies or music stored in on hard drives or iPads (**Fig. 14**). Inside the operating room (see **Fig. 14**), patients usually enjoy watching movies or listening to music with earphones during surgery. They are placed in a reclining position, extending the hand for the surgeons to operate on (**Figs. 15** and **16**). This transforms the patient's experience from potentially psychologically stressful surgery into a movie-theater experience (see **Fig. 15**). Many patients have told surgeons that they had a great experience in the operating room.

More surgical observers and trainees can be allowed in the operating room for teaching purposes because the procedures do not involve anesthesiologists and their equipment. In China, wide-awake hand operations are not typically performed in a minor procedure room. The operating room is usually large, similar to that of an ordinary operating room, but the regulations are slightly less stringent because the operations are usually simpler than complex reconstruction.

In general, the wide-awake approach increases the efficiency of departmental workflow, offers more room for surgical observers, and decreases the load on major operating rooms, allowing other departments to arrange urgent operations more easily. The entire hospital benefits from less pressure in allotting anesthesiologists and reserving surgical recovery rooms, which typically can become a nightmare on certain busy days or seasons of the year. By establishing this operating room close to surgeons' offices, surgeons save a huge amount of time and labor.

FUTURE PERSPECTIVES

Chinese hand surgeons have adopted wide-awake hand surgical approaches quickly in treating a variety of hand disorders. Because of the diverse landscape of the country, surgeons working in more inland areas have not yet begun to use this approach. Nevertheless, the authors expect the popularity of this technique to increase in those hospitals in the near future. Chinese hand surgeons have already organized 2

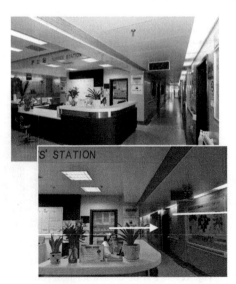
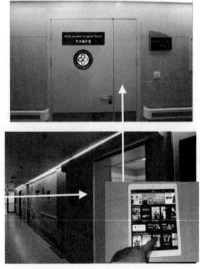

Fig. 14. The location and setting of the wide-awake surgical room (*top left*). From the nurse station (*bottom left*), patient may pick up a favorite movie (*bottom right*), before going into the room (*top right*).

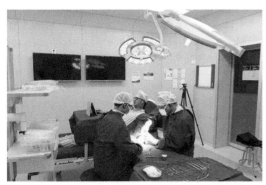

Fig. 15. The inside view of the new wide-awake hand surgery room in Nantong University.

courses and a congress symposium on this topic; through these efforts this technique has been popularized quickly. Feedback from the attendees is very positive; Chinese hand surgeons seem to have less resistance to this technique than has been seen in some other countries. The experience in China demonstrates that this is a safe method; no complications from use of epinephrine have been reported. The authors estimate that about 100 hand surgeons in China now regularly use this method; 10 hospitals report regular use. In addition, a book was published this year on this technique, based on the experience of 6 units. The authors expect further popularization in the next few years. Chinese

patients are very willing to undergo surgeries in that setting. The administrative system also welcomes the new approach because it benefits the hospital, surgeons, and patients through improved efficiency in treatment and better distribution of resources, as well as savings in materials and cost.

REFERENCES

1. Lalonde DH, Wong A. Dosage of local anesthesia in wide awake hand surgery. J Hand Surg Am 2013;38: 2025–8.
2. Lalonde DH. Wide-awake flexor tendon repair. Plast Reconstr Surg 2009;123:623–5.
3. Lalonde D, Higgins A. Wide awake flexor tendon repair in the finger. Plast Reconstr Surg Glob Open 2016;4:e797.
4. Lalonde DH. Reconstruction of the hand with wide awake surgery. Clin Plast Surg 2011;38: 761–9.
5. Lalonde D. Minimally invasive anesthesia in wide awake hand surgery. Hand Clin 2014;30:1–6.
6. Liodaki E, Xing SG, Mailaender P, et al. Management of difficult intra-articular fractures or fracture dislocations of the proximal interphalangeal joint. J Hand Surg Eur Vol 2015;40:16–23.
7. Liverneaux PA, Ichihara S, Hendriks S, et al. Fractures and dislocation of the base of the thumb metacarpal. J Hand Surg Eur Vol 2015; 40:42–50.
8. Tang JB. Efficient and elaborate treatment of hand fractures. J Hand Surg Eur Vol 2015;40:7.
9. Wada T, Oda T. Mallet fingers with bone avulsion and DIP joint subluxation. J Hand Surg Eur Vol 2015;40:8–15.
10. Shewring DJ, Miller AC, Ghandour A. Condylar fractures of the proximal and middle phalanges. J Hand Surg Eur Vol 2015;40:51–8.
11. Tang JB, Blazar PE, Giddins G, et al. Overview of indications, preferred methods and technical tips for hand fractures from around the world. J Hand Surg Eur Vol 2015;40:88–9.
12. Batdorf NJ, Cantwell SR, Moran SL. Idiopathic carpal tunnel syndrome in children and adolescents. J Hand Surg Am 2015;40:773–7.
13. Cho YJ, Lee JH, Shin DJ, et al. Comparison of short wrist transverse open and limited open techniques for carpal tunnel release: a randomized controlled trial of two incisions. J Hand Surg Eur Vol 2016;41:143–7.
14. Lee LH, Al-Maiyah M, Al-Bahrani RZ, et al. Outcome of carpal tunnel release–correlation with wrist and wrist-palm anthropomorphic measurements. J Hand Surg Eur Vol 2015;40:186–92.
15. Xing SG, Tang JB. Entrapment neuropathy of the wrist, forearm, and elbow. Clin Plast Surg 2014;41: 561–88.

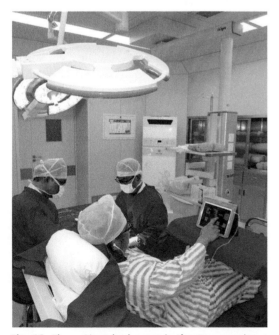

Fig. 16. The patient had a movie-theater experience during surgery, watching movie during surgery.

16. Tang JB, Amadio PC, Boyer MI, et al. Current practice of primary flexor tendon repair: a global view. Hand Clin 2013;29:179–89.

17. Tang JB. Wide-awake primary flexor tendon repair, tenolysis, and tendon transfer. Clin Orthop Surg 2015;7:275–81.

18. Lalonde DH, Martin AL. Wide-awake flexor tendon repair and early tendon mobilization in zones 1 and 2. Hand Clin 2013;29:207–13.

19. Tang JB. Indications, methods, postoperative motion and outcome evaluation of primary flexor tendon repairs in Zone 2. J Hand Surg Eur Vol 2007;32: 118–29.

20. Tang JB. Release of the A4 pulley to facilitate zone II flexor tendon repair. J Hand Surg Am 2014;39:2300–7.

21. Tang JB. Outcomes and evaluation of flexor tendon repair. Hand Clin 2013;29:251–9.

22. Zhou X, Li XR, Qing J, et al. Outcomes of the six-strand M-Tang repair for zone 2 primary flexor tendon repair in 54 fingers. J Hand Surg Eur Vol 2017;42:462–8.

23. Elliot D, Lalonde DH, Tang JB. Commentaries on clinical results of releasing the entire A2 pulley after flexor tendon repair in zone 2C. K. Moriya, T. Yoshizu, N. Tsubokawa, H. Narisawa, K. Hara and Y. Maki. J Hand Surg Eur. 2016, 41: 822-28. J Hand Surg Eur Vol 2016;41:829–30.

24. Rigo IZ, Røkkum M. Predictors of outcome after primary flexor tendon repair in zone 1, 2 and 3. J Hand Surg Eur Vol 2016;41:793–801.

25. Moriya K, Yoshizu T, Tsubokawa N, et al. Outcomes of release of the entire A4 pulley after flexor tendon repairs in zone 2A followed by early active mobilization. J Hand Surg Eur Vol 2016;41: 400–5.

26. Moriya K, Yoshizu T, Maki Y, et al. Clinical outcomes of early active mobilization following flexor tendon repair using the six-strand technique: short- and long-term evaluations. J Hand Surg Eur Vol 2015; 40:250–8.

27. Nicoson MC, Moran SL. Diagnosis and treatment of acute lunotriquetral ligament injuries. Hand Clin 2015;31:467–76.

28. Bednar JM. Acute Scapholunate ligament injuries: arthroscopic treatment. Hand Clin 2015;31: 417–23.

29. Lindau TR. The role of arthroscopy in carpal instability. J Hand Surg Eur Vol 2016;41:35–47.

30. Koehler SM, Guerra SM, Kim JM, et al. Outcome of arthroscopic reduction association of the scapholunate joint. J Hand Surg Eur Vol 2016;41: 48–55.

31. van de Grift TC, Ritt MJ. Management of lunotriquetral instability: a review of the literature. J Hand Surg Eur Vol 2016;41:72–85.

32. Xie RG, Xing SG, Tang JB. New procedures for precisely establishing volar wrist arthroscopic portals. J Hand Surg Eur Vol 2015;40:1014–5.

33. Hagert E, Lalonde DH. Wide-awake wrist arthroscopy and open TFCC repair. J Wrist Surg 2012;1: 55–60.

34. Tosti R, Shin E. Wrist arthroscopy for athletic injuries. Hand Clin 2017;33:107–17.

35. Desai MJ, Kamal RN, Richard MJ. Management of intercarpal ligament injuries associated with distal radius fractures. Hand Clin 2015;31:409–16.

Microsurgical Flaps in Repair and Reconstruction of the Hand

Shimpei Ono, MD, PhD[a],*,
Sandeep J. Sebastin, MCh (Plastic Surgery)[b], Hiroyuki Ohi, MD[c],
Kevin C. Chung, MD, MS[d]

KEYWORDS

- Hand • Soft tissue • Perforator flaps • Propeller flaps • Intrinsic hand flaps

KEY POINTS

- The authors have classified soft-tissue defects of the hand based on 3 criteria, namely the size of the defect, the location of the defect, and tissue characteristics.
- If the defect is small, primary closure or conventional local flap is preferred. Larger defects require distant or free flaps. Pedicle perforator flaps are a good choice for medium-sized defects.
- Flap reconstruction should take into consideration functional aesthetic units and subunits of the hand and skin incision lines, and the flap's border should be placed along skin creases and/or mid-lateral lines of the digits and hand.
- Like-with-like reconstruction is preferable, because palmar and dorsal skin have different functional and aesthetic characteristics.

INTRODUCTION

Early coverage of soft-tissue defects of the hand following trauma or tumor resection with well-vascularized flaps can provide an excellent functional outcome. It protects underlying structures such as bone, joint, tendon, nerves, and vessels, and brings in additional nourishment to the wound bed. Minimal scarring and early rehabilitation prevent tendon adhesion and/or joint stiffness. The goal of soft-tissue coverage of the hand has traditionally focused on restoring hand function. However, recent studies based on patient-reported outcomes have shown that aesthetic concerns are equally important. An improvement in appearance of the hand is an important factor for patients with hand deformities seeking reconstructive hand surgery.[1–3] This improves patients' quality of life.[4–6] The focus of soft-tissue coverage of the hand has shifted from simply closing the defect to achieving a functional as well as an aesthetic outcome.

Advances in perforator flaps enable surgeons to harvest thin, pliable, and well-vascularized cutaneous flaps with minimal donor-site morbidity by preserving the underlying muscle and the possibility of linear closure of the donor defect rather than skin grafting. Perforator flaps may be raised as free flaps or pedicle flaps. Free perforator flaps, which are harvested from remote sites, are useful in resurfacing larger defects, but the aesthetic outcome may not be ideal owing to differences in tissue characteristics. On the other hand, pedicle perforator flaps can provide superior aesthetic

The authors have nothing to disclose.
[a] Department of Plastic, Reconstructive and Aesthetic Surgery, Nippon Medical School, 1-1-5 Sendagi, Bunkyo-ku, Tokyo 113-8603, Japan; [b] Department of Hand and Reconstructive Microsurgery, National University Health System, Singapore, Singapore; [c] Hand & Microsurgery Center, Seirei Hamamatsu General Hospital, Shizuoka, Japan; [d] Section of Plastic Surgery, Department of Surgery, The University of Michigan Health System, Ann Arbor, MI, USA
* Corresponding author.
E-mail address: s-ono@nms.ac.jp

Hand Clin 33 (2017) 425–441
http://dx.doi.org/10.1016/j.hcl.2017.04.001

outcomes, because defects are covered with similar tissue from adjacent locations based on the principle of replacing like-with-like. Therefore, it is important to expand the indications for pedicle perforator flaps in reconstruction of the hand. The aim of this article is to present the authors' strategy of cutaneous coverage of the hand with a focus on perforator flaps.

CLASSIFICATION OF SOFT-TISSUE DEFECTS

Soft-tissue defects of the hand can be classified based on the size of the defect (small, medium, and large), the location of the defect (distal finger [tip to proximal interphalangeal joint, PIPJ], proximal finger [PIPJ to metacarpophalangeal joint, MCPJ], and hand [MCPJ to wrist]) and tissue characteristics (dorsal and palmar).

Defects can be classified based on size into small, medium, and large (**Fig. 1**). It is important to understand that this classification is subjective and based on the anatomic site. Instead of considering size as a number, such as 3 cm in diameter, the authors feel it is more useful to relate size to an anatomic feature. For digits, if the defect is restricted to 1 surface (dorsal, palmar, lateral, or Web space) of a phalanx, it is considered as a small defect. If it extends to 2 adjacent surfaces of a phalanx or it involves 1 surface of 2 adjacent phalanges, it is considered as a medium-sized defect. All other defects (eg, more than 2 surfaces of a phalanx, 1 surface of 3 phalanges, defects on multiple fingers, noncontiguous defects on a single finger) are considered as large defects. Similarly, for the hand, if the defect is restricted to 1 surface of a single metacarpal (dorsal, palmar, lateral or web-space), it is considered as a small defect. If it involves 2 adjacent surfaces of a single metacarpal or 2 adjacent metacarpals, it is considered as a medium-sized defect. All other defects (eg, more than 2 surfaces of a single metacarpal, more than 2 metacarpals, noncontiguous defects) are considered as large defects.

Defects can also be classified based on location. This is based on the concept of functional cutaneous units of the hand introduced by Tubiana.[7] He divided the hand into several functional units taking into account mobility versus stability of the hand. The lines separating the units were traditionally used for surgical skin incisions, permitting access while minimizing scar contracture. In 2015, Rehim and colleagues[8] modified Tubiana's concept and introduced functional aesthetic units and subunits of the hand, taking into consideration the principles of visual

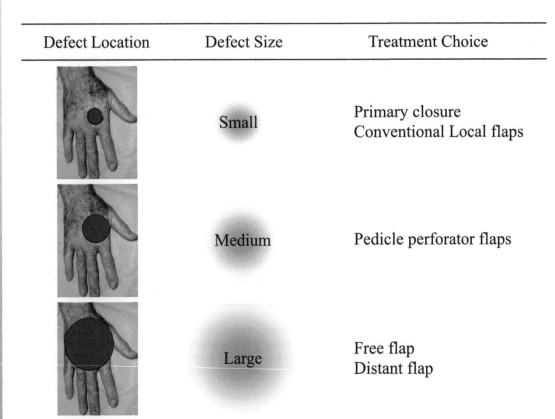

Defect Location	Defect Size	Treatment Choice
	Small	Primary closure Conventional Local flaps
	Medium	Pedicle perforator flaps
	Large	Free flap Distant flap

Fig. 1. Preferred treatment choices based on size and location of defects.

perception as well as the topographic and anatomic features of the hand. The current authors have modified Rehim and colleagues' functional aesthetic units to make it simpler to classify soft-tissue defects of the hand (**Fig. 2**). In essence, there are 3 functional aesthetic units, 2 for the digits (distal finger or distal thumb and proximal finger or proximal thumb), and 1 for the hand. The distal finger or thumb unit extends from the tip to the PIPJ of the finger or interphalangeal joint (IPJ) of the thumb and the proximal finger or thumb unit extends from the PIPJ/IPJ to the MCPJ. The hand unit extends from the MCPJ to the wrist.

Defects can also be classified based on tissue characteristics into dorsal and palmar defects. The characteristics of the palmar and dorsal skin of the hand are very different, which is aesthetically and functionally relevant. The skin on the palmar side is thick, hairless, and immobile, because the skin is attached to the underlying palmar aponeurosis by numerous vertical fibers, facilitating grasp. The dorsal skin, on the other hand, is thin, supple, and quite mobile due to loose areolar tissue, which accommodates to the extremes of digital flexion and extension.

Overall, reconstruction of soft-tissue defects of the hand can be considered under the following headings:

1. Distal finger/thumb unit
   a. Dorsal (small, medium, large)
   b. Palmar (small, medium, large)
2. Proximal finger/thumb unit
   a. Dorsal (small, medium, large)
   b. Palmar (small, medium, large)
3. Hand unit
   a. Dorsal (small, medium, large)
   b. Palmar (small, medium, large)

OUR STRATEGY OF HAND COVERAGE

Various flaps have been described to cover soft-tissue defects of the hand. However, it is still challenging to choose the right flap that will provide the best functional and aesthetic outcome for a particular defect. This is because multiple factors need to be considered.[9] These factors include characteristics of the defect (size, location, and depth), characteristics of the flap (color, texture, thickness, hairiness, sensitivity, reliability, donor site morbidity), patient characteristics (age, sex, handedness, occupation, and comorbid conditions), and surgeon factors (knowledge, experience, and microsurgical ability).

If the defect is small, primary closure and conventional local flaps (advancement, transposition, or rotation flaps) are good treatment options, providing immediate closure, rapid healing time, and an excellent aesthetic result. On the other hand, large defects require free or distant flaps although the skin color, texture, and thickness match are often not ideal. For medium-sized

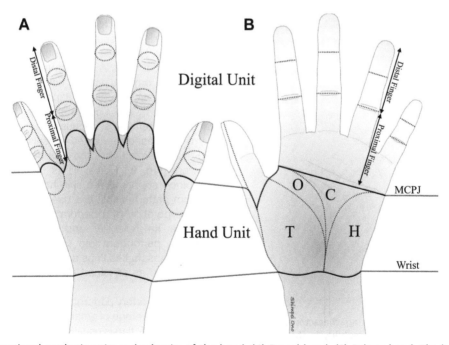

Fig. 2. Functional aesthetic units and subunits of the hand. (*A*) Dorsal hand. (*B*) Palmar hand. The hand palm can be considered as a single functional aesthetic unit that is further subdivided into 4 subunits; Thenar (T), Opposition (O), Hypothenar (H), and Central triangular (C). (*Courtesy of* S. Ono, MD, PhD, Tokyo, Japan.)

defects, the authors believe pedicle perforator flaps, especially propeller designs, represent a good choice. Unlike the trunk, there is a limited amount of skin in the transverse axis of the extremities (**Fig. 3**). However, the extremities have a tapering diameter allowing one to transfer skin raised in the longitudinal axis from proximal to distal. A propeller design perforator flap takes advantage of this anatomic characteristic. In the upper limb, a perforator-based propeller flap is based on a perforator proximal to a defect and designed as an asymmetric propeller. This allows the larger limb of the asymmetric propeller after rotation through 180° around its vascular axis to cover the primary defect and the shorter limb to contribute toward primary closure of the secondary defect[10] (**Fig. 4**).

The authors believe in replacing like with like. They prefer to use a dorsal flap for dorsal defects and a palmar flap for palmar defects. Larger defects may require a free flap. Although many free flap choices are available for large dorsal defects, the foot remains the only source of glabrous skin. The toe pulp flap can be used to resurface digital pulp defects, whereas the instep flap can provide a larger area of tissue, approaching the size of an entire palmar finger or a comparable palmar defect. Similarly when skin grafting is considered for the primary or the secondary defect, tone must consider unique hand characteristics again.

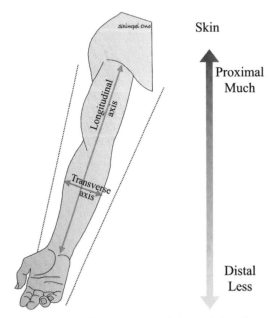

Fig. 3. Schema demonstrating characteristics of extremities with limited skin mobility in the transverse axis, and tapered shape that allows transfer of skin raised in the longitudinal axis from proximal to distal. (*Courtesy of* S. Ono, MD, PhD, Tokyo, Japan.)

Skin grafts transferred from the thenar or hypothenar eminences or plantar instep to the palmar provide better skin match (**Fig. 5**). Skin grafts from the forearm to palmar defects, even from the volar forearm to the palm, result in poorer aesthetic results. The characteristics of the palmar hand are totally different from the dorsal hand and volar/dorsal forearm (**Fig. 6**). For dorsal hand and/or finger defects, our preferred donor-sites of skin grafting are proximal forearm, particularly from the medial aspect. The other choice is the dorsolateral aspects of the hand, over the first or fifth metacarpal bones, where the donor site can be closed primarily by advancing the dorsolateral skin margins toward the midlateral line, leaving the postoperative scar in the desirable midlateral line.

FLAP SELECTION BASED ON DEFECT SIZE AND LOCATION

The authors' preferred flap selection based on defects size and location is summarized in **Fig. 7** (dorsal side) and **Fig. 8** (palmar side).

Distal Finger Unit (from Fingertip to PIPJ)

Dorsal finger

Dorsal finger defects distal to the PIPJ should ideally be covered with dorsal finger/hand tissue based on replacing like with like. The distal subunit of the digit is unique in appearance because of the nail. If patients desire restoration of their nail complex, a nail transfer from their toe, such as partial-toe transfer[11] or vascularized nail transfer,[12] is the only choice. However, these options demand high microsurgical skills. A small defect in this region, less than 1 cm in diameter, can be covered with local flaps, such as bilobe flaps or rotation flaps. Local flaps are conventionally considered random-pattern flaps, because their vascular supply is not based on named vessels. Rather, they are vascularized by the subdermal vascular network (**Fig. 9**). However, as understanding of the blood supply to the skin has improved, true random-pattern flaps are used less frequently, as incorporation of a perforator into the flap will increase its reliability and dimensions. Thus, including perforators into conventional random-pattern flaps makes flaps safer and enables them to be raised as an island allowing additional flap reach.

The digital artery perforator (DAP) flap is a useful option for coverage of small to medium digital defects. The DAP flap is usually designed on the dorsal skin over the middle phalanx and vascularized by perforating branches of the digital artery running from the palmar to the dorsal side of the

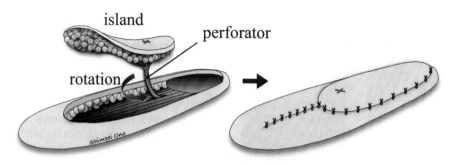

island

perforator

rotation

Shimpei Ono

Perforator-based propeller flaps

Fig. 4. Demonstration of a perforator-based propeller design flap. (*Courtesy of* S. Ono, MD, PhD, Tokyo, Japan.)

finger. These are the same branches that nourish the traditional cross-finger flap. One may design the DAP flap on the dorsal skin over the proximal phalanx and be able to cover a dorsal defect beyond the PIPJ by rotating the flap from proximal to distal. Some authors have reported use of the DAP flap for fingertip and pulp reconstruction,[13] but the current authors prefer to use this flap for dorsal digital defects. This allows reconstruction of defects using similar tissue and reduction of the rotation of the perforator pedicle to less than 90°. The DAP flap can be designed as an ellipse shape and can range from 1 to 2 cm in length and 1 cm in width for a cutaneous flap design.[14] The secondary defect after a DAP flap usually requires a skin graft.

The reverse cross-finger flap can also be considered for medium-sized dorsal digital defects.[15] However, this requires a second procedure to divide the flap and has the potential to cause joint stiffness, especially in elderly patients. The application of artificial dermis and subsequent skin grafting may be a more appealing option in the elderly, as patients are able to move their finger immediately after surgery. For medium-to-large-sized dorsal defects, a distant pedicle flap from other anatomic sites (eg, abdominal or groin flap) is still a versatile and reliable option to save the affected finger, although disadvantages include the need for staged operations, the bulk of the flap with subsequent debulking, and poorer aesthetic outcomes. The authors prefer to use

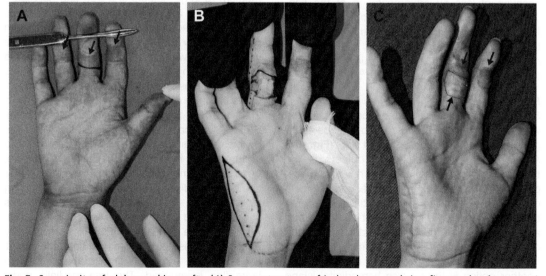

Fig. 5. Superiority of glabrous skin grafts. (*A*) Scar contracture of index, long, and ring fingers that have previously undergone release and full-thickness skin grafts from the groin. (*B*) Application of full-thickness skin graft harvested from the hypothenar region. (*C*) Superior color match of hypothenar FTSG (*black arrow*) to groin FTSG (*blue arrows*).

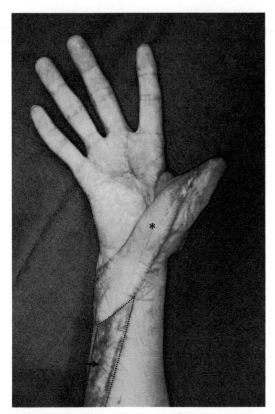

Fig. 6. Poor aesthetic appearance after reconstruction of a palmar defect using a nonglabrous skin flap (ulnar artery perforator-based propeller flap). *Black Asterisk*: Flap harvested from forearm. *Black arrow*: Flap donor-site.

pedicle abdominal flaps rather than groin flaps because of less hyperpigmentation of the flap. When harvesting the pedicle abdominal flap, the flap is primarily thinned down to the layer where the subdermal vascular network can be seen through a minimal fat layer, to achieve good contour reconstruction of the fingers.[16]

Palmar finger

Small size distal palmar defects can be covered with a V-Y advancement flap and oblique triangular neurovascular advancement flap (**Fig. 10**). Another option for small-sized defects is the thenar flap. It is a reasonable and reliable choice, particularly in the index and long fingers. Defects can be covered using a similar tissue from the thenar eminence. The finger is left attached, and after 2 to 3 weeks the flap is divided. The major disadvantage of this flap is the possibility of PIPJ flexion contracture, especially in older patients. Another option is the reverse homodigital island flap (**Fig. 11**). This is a single-stage procedure; maintaining the middle transverse digital palmar arch intact is the most important factor for flap

viability. The common complications of this flap include cold intolerance, venous congestion, and flexion contracture of the PIPJ.[17] To prevent venous congestion of the flap, the flap pedicle should be raised with a generous cuff of subcutaneous fat tissue to create venous drainage from the tiny perivascular venules. Some authors have reported excellent functional and aesthetic outcomes of fingertip reconstruction with partial medial second toe pulp free flaps.[18] This flap requires a high level of microsurgical skill, which may not always be feasible or available. Additionally, donor site morbidity may be significant. Free or distant tissue transfers should be considered in medium- and large-sized defects. For medium-sized defects of the fingers involving more than 1 phalangeal segment, the heterodigital artery island flap is a reliable method of reconstruction. This flap is an island flap typically raised from the ulnar aspect of the long or ring fingers, although most surgeons prefer the long finger, because the pedicle is longer, based on the ulnar digital artery, and the venae comitantes. Unlike the neurovascular island flap, the digital nerve is left in situ in the donor finger, thus avoiding neurologic complications. This flap has several advantages, such as the possibility of one-staged operation, easy postoperative mobilization with good functional recovery, and satisfactory aesthetic results. The disadvantages include the sacrifice of the common digital artery, as well as the need to violate an uninjured healthy finger, and poor aesthetic results of the donor site after skin grafting. Another option to reconstruct medium-to-large defects is a free flap harvested from the volar aspect of the wrist (**Fig. 12**). This flap is nourished by the superficial palmar branch of radial artery (SPBRA). It is designed over the volar aspect with an elliptical shape, with the main axis along the wrist crease that facilitates donor site closure.[19] The SPBRA usually bifurcates from the main trunk of the radial artery 1 to 2 cm proximal to the distal wrist crease.[20,21] The SPBRA flap has several advantages; it is thin, pliable, and hairless, resulting in a nice color and texture match in covering palmar finger defects, up to 50 × 25 mm in size. The postoperative donor site scar is indistinguishable from the preexisting wrist creases. Additionally, no major vessel is sacrificed, and only 1 operative field is required. Although the SPBRA flap is technically demanding, it is one of the useful flaps for palmar finger defects. If multiple fingers are involved, a large flap is required. The free medialis pedis flap, which is outlined on the medial border of the foot, is recommended for functional and aesthetic reasons based on the from foot-to-

Defect Location	Defect Size	Treatment Choice
● From fingertip to PIPJ 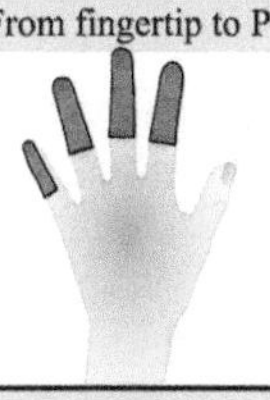	Small	Primary closure, Conventional local flap DAP flap
	Medium	DAP flap Reverse cross-finger flap (Younger) Artificial dermis with skin graft (Elder)
	Large	Distant flap (eg, Pedicle thin abdominal flap)
● From PIPJ to MCPJ 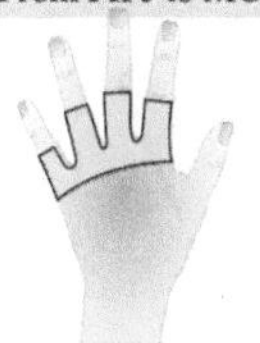	Small	Primary closure, Conventional local flap DMAP flap Flag flap, Axial flag flap, Reverse cross-finger flap
	Medium to Large	Retrograde flow flap (eg, Radial forearm flap, PIA flap) Free flap (eg, Dorsalis pedis flap, ALT flap) Distant flap (eg, Pedicle thin abdominal flap)
● From MCPJ to Wrist 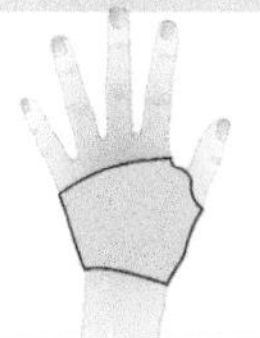	Small	Primary closure, Conventional local flap
	Medium	RAP flap (radial side), UAP flap (ulnar side) PIA flap
	Large	Free flap (eg, Dorsalis pedis flap, ALT flap) Distant flap (eg, Pedicle thin abdominal flap)
● Dorsal thumb 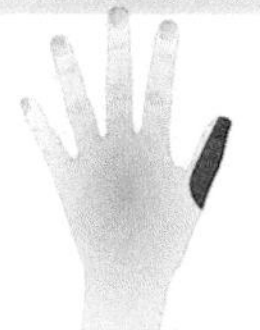	Small	Primary closure, Conventional local flap Reverse homodigital dorsoradial/dorsoulnar flaps
	Medium	FDMA flap
	Large	Free flap (eg, Dorsalis pedis flap) RAP flap, PIA flap

Fig. 7. Choice of flaps based on size and location of defects (dorsal side).

Defect Location	Defect Size	Treatment Choice
● From fingertip to PIPJ 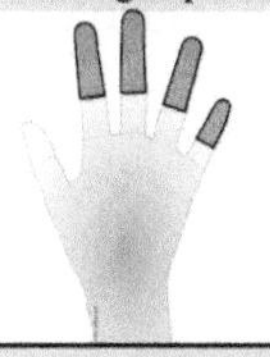	Small	Secondary intension (if bone is not exposed) V-Y advancement flap, Oblique triangular flap Thenar flap (Younger), Homodigital island flap Toe pulp free flap
	Medium to Large	Heterodigital island flap Free flap (SPBRA flap, Mediais pedis flap)
● From PIPJ to MCPJ 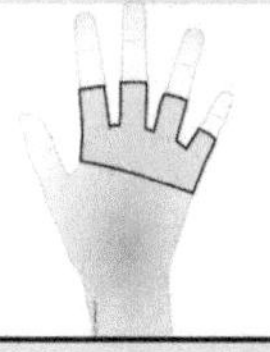	Small	Primary closure, Conventional local flap Heterodigital island flap
	Medium	Free flap (SPBRA flap, Medialis pedis flap) Axial flag flap, Cross-finger flap
	Large	Free flap (eg, Medialis pedis flap, ALT flap) Distant flap (eg, Pedicle thin abdominal flap)
● From MCPJ to Wrist 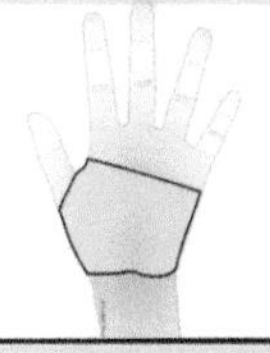	Small	Conventional local flap Secondary intension (if vital structures are not exposed)
	Medium-to-Large	Free medialis pedis flap Free flap (eg, ALT flap) Distant flap (eg, Pedicle thin abdominal flap)
● Palmar thumb 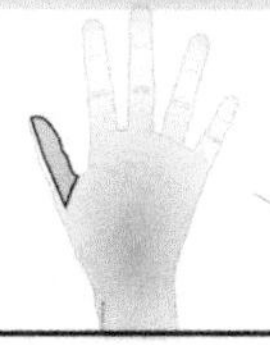	Small	Moberg advancement flap
	Medium	Heterodigital island flap Toe pulp free flap
	Large	Free medialis pedis flap Distant flap (eg, Pedicle thin abdominal flap)

Fig. 8. Choice of flaps based on size and location of defects (palmar side).

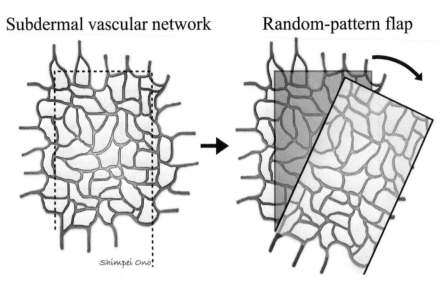

Subdermal vascular network   Random-pattern flap

Shimpei Ono

Fig. 9. Vascular basis of random-pattern flaps. (*Courtesy of* S. Ono, MD, PhD, Tokyo, Japan.)

hand concept. The free flap from the medial plantar region has several advantages. It provides good color, texture, and thickness matching for palmar hand/finger resurfacing (**Fig. 13**); it can be used as a flow-through flap; and the size of pedicle vessels is compatible with the recipient vessels in the hand/finger. Additionally, it consists of glabrous skin rich in nerve endings, so it has good potential for sensory recovery. Usually, the flap is designated to cover all defects of involved

fingers to form mitten hand at the initial operation, and the surgical syndactyly is separated several months later.

Proximal Finger Unit

Dorsal defect

Small defects can be covered with the dorsal metacarpal artery perforator (DMAP) flap (**Fig. 14**). The DMAP flap was introduced by Quaba in 1990

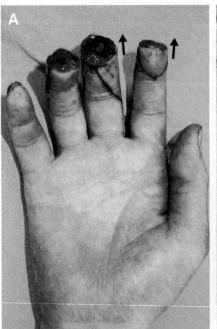
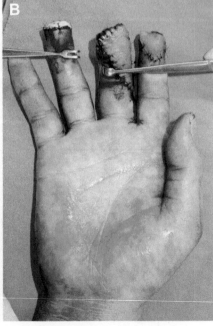

Fig. 10. Use of a V-Y advancement flap and an oblique triangular neurovascular island flap for reconstruction of small size pulp defect in the index and long fingers, respectively. (*A*) Flap design. (*B*) After flap advancement. *Black arrow* indicates direction of flap advancement.

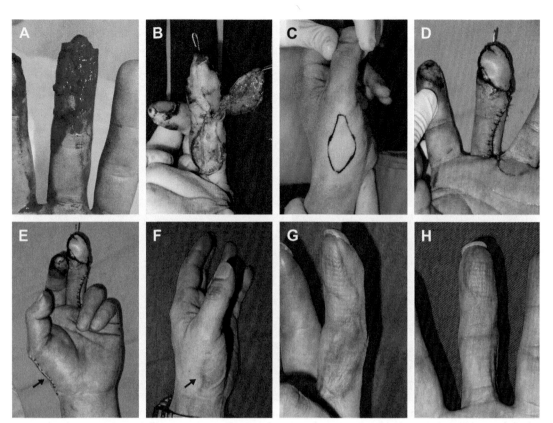

Fig. 11. Design, transfer and outcome of a reverse vascular island flap for a small-sized digital pulp defect. (*A*) Finger defect. (*B*) Flap harvesting.(*C*) Full-thickness skin grafts from the thenar area. (*D, E*) Immediate post-op. (*F–H*) Post-op 6 months. *Black arrow* indicates donor-site of skin graft.

as a distally based dorsal hand flap.[22] This flap is based on a perforator arising from the second, third, or fourth dorsal metacarpal artery (DMA) at the level of the metacarpal neck immediately distal to the juncturae tendinae (**Fig. 15**).[22,23] A preoperative Doppler assessment is not required, because the perforator is always present. In cases where the DMA is absent, the perforator arises directly from the deep palmar metacarpal artery. The flap is typically designed as an elliptical shape with the proximal limit defined by the distal edge of the extensor retinaculum, the distal limit as the metacarpal head, and the lateral border of adjoining metacarpals as the lateral limits (**Fig. 16**). This flap can be rotated 180° around a perforator and cover the dorsal and lateral finger soft tissue defects up to over the PIPJ safely. This flap can cover not only the finger dorsum defects but also palmar defects; however, the authors prefer to use this flap for finger dorsal (and/or lateral) coverage. Closure of the flap donor site on the hand dorsum may result in a visible scar. Thus, management of intraoperative and postoperative scarring is essential to improve the postsurgical scar aesthetically, which includes absorbable sutures in the deep

dermis to reduce skin tension, providing adhesive taping to reduce skin tension, and compression to prevent hypertrophic scar formation. The flag flap, axial flag flaps, and the reverse cross-finger flap from adjacent finger dorsum are alternative secondary options, but there are several disadvantages, including staged operations and a skin graft for the donor site resulting in a poor aesthetic appearance. Medium- and large-sized defects in this region can be covered with a pedicle radial forearm flap, posterior interosseous artery (PIA) flap, distant pedicle flaps (eg, abdominal flap) or free flaps (eg, anterolateral thigh flap, ALT flap). Some authors reported use of the dorsalis pedis free flap for dorsal hand/finger reconstruction.[24] This flap can be harvested to contain various tissues including bone, joint, and tendon, and is particularly useful to reconstruct composite hand defects. The dorsalis pedis free flap is one of the best flaps based on this concept that provide a highly desirable color–texture match to dorsal hand/finger skin. Although significant donor site morbidity has been recognized previously, recent reports have documented fewer donor site problems. Further studies are

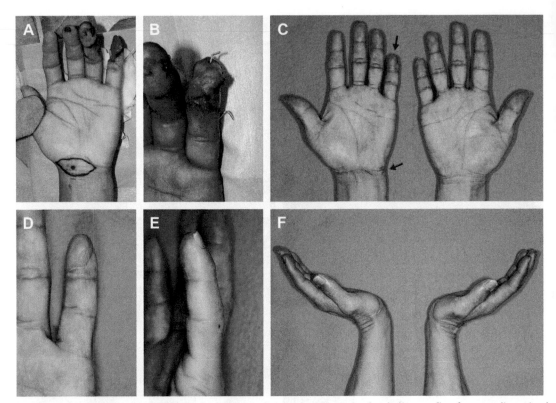

Fig. 12. Design, transfer and outcome of a free superficial palmar branch of radial artery flap for a medium-sized pulp defect. (*A*) Flap design. (*B*) After flap transfer. (*C–E*) Post-op 6 months view. (*F*) No restriction of wrist extension. *Black arrow* indicates transfered flap. *Blue arrow* indicates flap donor-site.

needed on this flap to evaluate the comprehensive long-term outcomes, including donor site morbidity.

Palmar defect

Small defects can be covered with heterodigital island flaps. The options for medium-sized defects include the SPBRA flap and free medialis pedis flap. When segmental digital artery defects are encountered, these flaps can be transposed as a flow-through flap to cover the skin defect and reconstruct the digital artery flow at the same time. Axial flag flaps and cross-finger flaps from the dorsum of an adjacent finger are safer choices, but should be limited in the cases for which free tissue transfer is not possible or not likely to succeed. Larger defects in this region are generally covered by free flaps (eg, medialis pedis flaps or ALT flaps) or distant flaps (eg, abdominal flap). The free medialis pedis flap is an ideal choice; however, there is a limitation of potential flap size; the maximum size is approximately 5 × 10 cm. Therefore, if the defect size exceeds this limitation, tone must choose the ALT flaps or distant thin abdominal flaps.

Thumb Defects

Dorsal defects

The reverse homodigital dorsoradial and dorsoulnar flaps are useful in resurfacing small dorsal thumb defects.[25,26] These flaps are supplied by the dorsoradial and dorsoulnar digital arteries, which arise from the radial artery at the level of the anatomic snuffbox, and the palmar arteries at the level of the head of the thumb metacarpal bone, respectively. They run on their respective sides to supply the skin over the dorsum of the thumb. When using these flaps as reverse flow flaps, the distal point of the vascular connection is important where there is usually a pivot point for flap rotation. Preservation of the connection is mandatory to ensure adequate blood supply to the flap. The dorsoradial digital artery has consistent connections with the palmar vascular system at the middle third of the proximal phalanx. On the other hand, the dorsoulnar digital artery has an anastomosis with the ulnar palmar digital artery at the neck of the proximal phalanx. These flaps are useful to cover the small-sized defect, and the flap donor-site can be closed primarily (**Fig. 17**). If both flaps are applicable to the defect, the dorsoradial flaps are preferred, because the

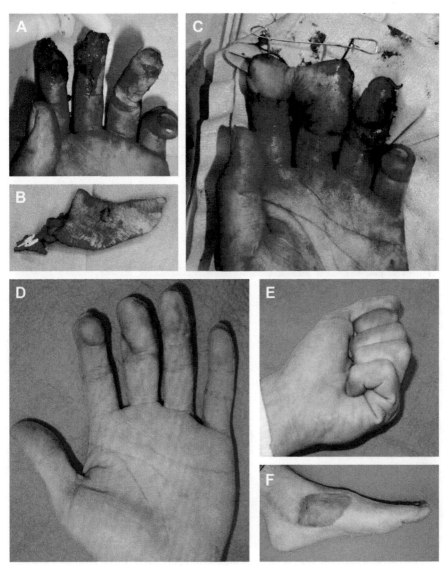

Fig. 13. Use of a free medialis pedis flap for a large-sized pulp defect involving multiple digits. (*A*) Index and long finger defects. (*B*) A free medialis pedis flap. (*C*) Immediate post-op. (*D–F*) Post-op 6 months.

dorsoulnar flaps have a potential risk of first Web contracture and reduced MCPJ motion for larger flaps, wider than 2 × 1 cm. For medium-sized dorsal thumb defects, the first dorsal metacarpal artery (FDMA) flap, also known as kite flap, is a good option. This flap is an island pedicle flap harvested from the dorsal surface of the index finger and based on the first dorsal metacarpal artery and venae comitantes. The FDMA flap is a versatile flap to cover the dorsal thumb defect; however, the disadvantages of the flap include creating a conspicuous donor site defect closed with a skin graft. Because this flap can be harvested as a sensate flap by including a branch of radial sensory nerve, some authors use this flap for palmar

thumb reconstruction. However, the authors rarely use dorsal hand/finger flaps for palmar thumb reconstruction for functional and aesthetic reasons. Large defects of the dorsal thumb require pedicle flaps like the radial artery forearm flap or the posterior interosseous artery flap, or free flaps such as the dorsalis pedis flap.

Palmar defects
Small defects located at the distal thumb can be covered with a Moberg advancement flap. It is the best choice to achieve good functional and aesthetic goals. The presence of the independent arterial supply to the dorsal thumb allows the palmar skin to be advanced with the palmar

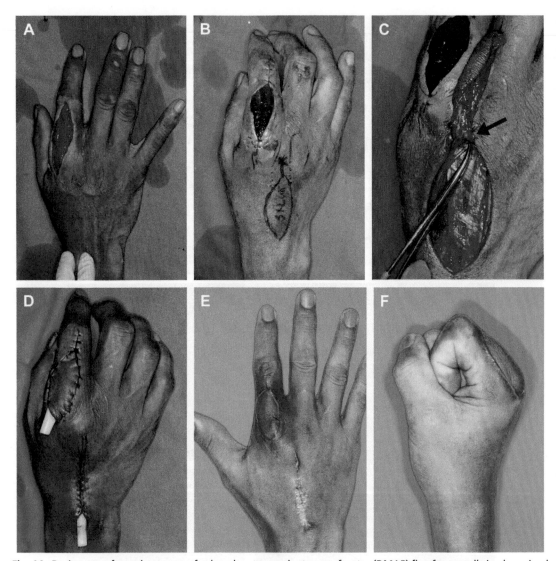

Fig. 14. Design, transfer and outcome of a dorsal metacarpal artery perforator (DMAP) flap for a small-sized proximal dorsal finger defect. (*A*) Dorsal finger defect. (*B*) Flap design. (*C*) *Black arrow* indicates perforator. (*D*) Immediate post-op. (*E, F*) Post-op 6 months. *Red cross* indicates the point where the perforator penetrates the deep fascia.

neurovascular bundles without sacrificing perfusion of the dorsal thumb skin. The major concern of the Moberg advancement flap is the potential risk of an IPJ flexion contracture because of the tension at

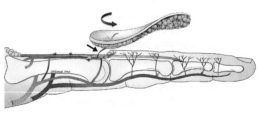

Fig. 15. Vascular anatomy of the dorsal metacarpal artery flap. *Black arrow*: the dorsal metacarpal artery perforator. *Blue arrow*: flap rotation around perforator. (*Courtesy of* S. Ono, MD, PhD, Tokyo, Japan.)

the closure site. To prevent IPJ flexion contracture, the proximal end of the flap can be modified to extend across the MCPJ crease as a V-shaped incision[27,28] or transverse incision along the MCPJ crease with a skin graft[29] to gain further distal flap advancement. Medium-sized defects can be covered with either a heterodigital island flap or a free toe pulp flap. Large defects require free or distant flaps; the free medialis pedis flap is one of the best choices to achieve good outcomes.

Hand Unit

Dorsal defects

Linear closure and conventional local flaps are good options for small-sized defects. The choices

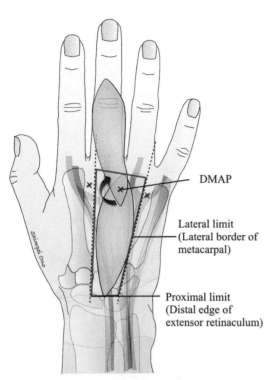

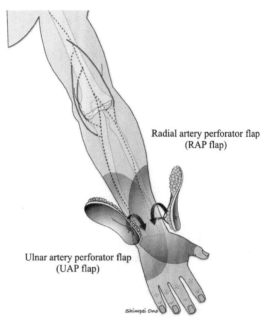

Fig. 16. Design and limits of the DMAP flap. (*Courtesy of* S. Ono, MD, PhD, Tokyo, Japan.)

Fig. 18. The arc of rotation of ulnar/radial artery perforator-based propeller flaps. (*Courtesy of* S. Ono, MD, PhD, Tokyo, Japan.)

for medium-sized defects include the radial artery perforator (RAP) flaps, the ulnar artery perforator (UAP) flap, or the PIA flaps. The former 2 flaps can be harvested as perforator-based propeller flaps and can cover radial and ulnar-side defects on the dorsal hand, respectively (**Fig. 18**). These flaps can cover not only dorsal hand defects but also palmar defects; however, the authors prefer to use them for dorsal defects. The reliable

perforator of the RAP flap is located 1 to 3 cm proximal to the radial styloid process; the potential flap size is 12 × 4 cm. It can reach up to the MCPJ (a border of the unit) after rotation of the flap.[10] In a similar way, the distal reliable UAP is located 4 to 6 cm proximal to pisiform bone; the potential flap size is 12 × 4 cm. It can reach up to the MCPJ (**Fig. 19**). The PIA flap can be harvested as a reverse PIA flap based on retrograde flow through the PIA via anastomosis with the dorsal branch of

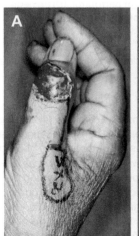
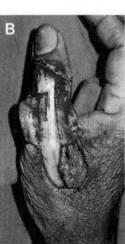
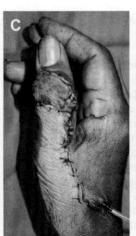
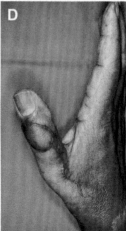

Fig. 17. Design, transfer and outcome of a thumb dorsoulnar flap for resurfacing small-size dorsal thumb defects. (*A*) Dorsal thumb defect and flap design. (*B*) Flap harvesting. (*C*) Immediate post-op. (*D*) Post-op 6 months.

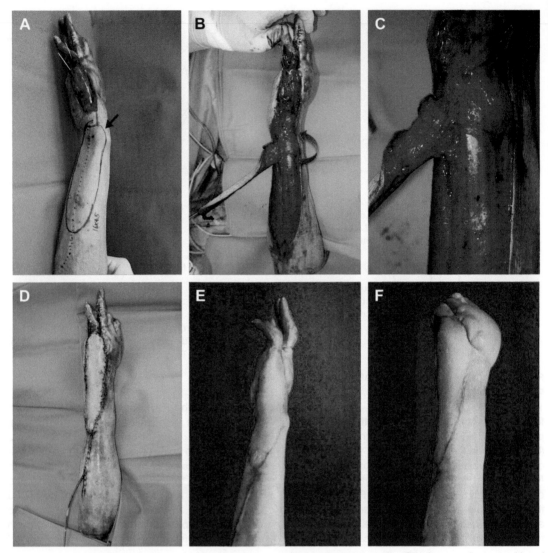

Fig. 19. Design, transfer and outcome of an ulnar artery perforator-based propeller flap for a medium-sized hand defect. (*A*) Dorsal hand defect and flap design. (*B*) Flap harvesting. (*C*) Enlarged view of perforator. (*D*) Immediate post-op. (*E, F*) Post-op 6 months. *Black arrow* indicates the point where the perforator penetrates the deep fascia.

the anterior interosseous artery and the dorsal carpal arterial arches near the wrist joint. The reverse PIA flap has traditionally been used to cover defects up to the MCPJ and for reconstruction of the first web space. The major drawbacks of the PIA flap include its anatomic variation (the PIA becomes very small as it runs distally in 6%[30] and the origin of the cutaneous perforator is located quite distally in 8%) and venous congestion. The use of pedicle flaps in cases with larger defects is more restricted. In particular the donor site appearance after harvesting a flap has been criticized because of long scars beyond the limits of the defect. Thus, for large defects, free flaps (eg, dorsalis pedis flap, ALT flap) (**Fig. 20**) or distant flaps (eg, pedicle thin abdominal flap) are recommended.

Palmar defects
Conventional local flaps can be considered for small defects in the palmar hand. Because the palm of the hand has a potential for healing secondarily, conservative treatments such as artificial dermis or healing by secondary intention may be good treatment options if deep vital structures are not exposed. For medium-sized defects, usefulness of the pedicle flaps harvested from the forearm, such as the RAP flap or UAP flap, are reported in the previous articles.[31–35] These flaps are thin and make it possible to reconstruct a good

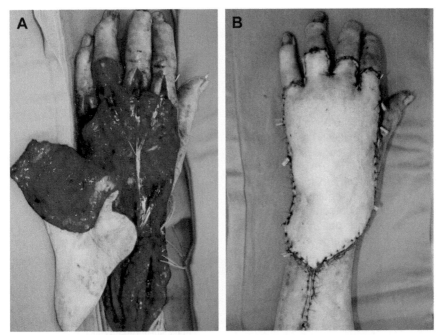

Fig. 20. (*A, B*) Outcomes of a free anterolateral thigh flap for a large-sized hand defect.

contour, however the aesthetic outcome is not good (see **Fig. 6**). Moreover, the reconstructed skin is not stable enough for the palmar region. The only available source of similar skin is the sole of the foot. Thus the authors prefer to use a free medialis pedis flap for replacing the weight-bearing areas of the palm. As described previously, because there is a limitation of flap size, larger defects require free or distant flap from other parts (**Fig. 21**).

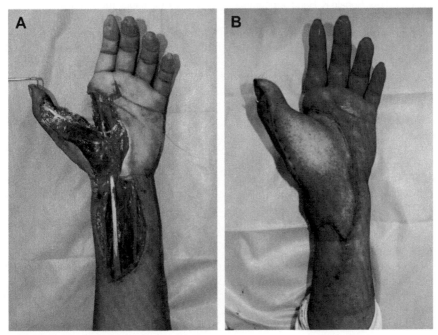

Fig. 21. (*A, B*) Aesthetic placement of an anterolateral thigh flap to resurface a large defect of the thumb and hand with attention to the functional units of the hand.

SUMMARY

The authors' strategy for soft-tissue coverage of the hand was presented. The concept of replacing like with like and reconstruction with similar adjacent tissue enhances both functional and aesthetic outcomes. In this viewpoint, the pedicle perforator flap is an ideal flap, particularly for medium-sized defects, but the donor site appearance after harvesting a relatively larger flap has been criticized because of longer scars beyond the limits of the defect. A decision-making algorithm to select an ideal flap for a particular hand defect is challenging, requiring experiential consideration of functional outcome, appearance, donor-site morbidity, and patient satisfaction. Recent efforts from Asian surgeons have been toward careful selection of the donor site and functional and cosmetic evaluation after flap transfer.[30,36–40] To assist surgeons in determining the most appropriate flap with more evidence, studies are necessary to compare the outcomes of each flap by evaluating hand function, aesthetics, donor site morbidity, and patient satisfaction.

REFERENCES

1. Chung KC, Kotsis SV, Kim HM, et al. Reasons why rheumatoid arthritis patients seek surgical treatment for hand deformities. J Hand Surg Am 2006;31:289–94.
2. Bogoch ER, Escott BG, Ronald K. Hand appearance as a patient motivation for surgery and a determinant of satisfaction with metacarpophalangeal joint arthroplasty for rheumatoid arthritis. J Hand Surg Am 2011;36:1007–14.
3. Bogoch ER, Judd MG. The hand: a second face? J Rheumatol 2002;29:2477–83.
4. Papadopulos NA, Kovacs L, Krammer S, et al. Quality of life following aesthetic plastic surgery: a prospective study. J Plast Reconstr Aesthet Surg 2007;60:915–21.
5. Von Soest T, Kvalem IL, Roald HE, et al. The effects of cosmetic surgery on body image, self-esteem, and psychological problems. J Plast Reconstr Aesthet Surg 2009;62:1238–44.
6. Kovacs L, Grob M, Zimmermann A, et al. Quality of life after severe hand injury. J Plast Reconstr Aesthet Surg 2011;64:1495–502.
7. Tubiana R. Functional anatomy: functional cutaneous units. In: Tubiana R, Thomine JM, Mackin E, editors. Examination of the hand and wrist. 2nd edition. London: Martin Dunitz; 1996. p. 145–6.
8. Rehim SA, Kowalski E, Chung KC. Enhancing aesthetic outcomes of soft-tissue coverage of the hand. Plast Reconstr Surg 2015;135:413e–28e.
9. Rehim SA, Chung KC. Local flaps of the hand. Hand Clin 2014;30:137–51.
10. Ono S, Sebastin SJ, Yazaki N, et al. Clinical applications of perforator based propeller flaps in upper limb soft tissue reconstruction. J Hand Surg Am 2011;36:853–63.
11. Koshima I, Inagawa K, Urushibara K, et al. Fingertip reconstructions using partial-toe transfers. Plast Reconstr Surg 2000;105:1666–74.
12. Endo T, Nakayama Y, Soeda S. Nail transfer: evolution of the reconstructive procedure. Plast Reconstr Surg 1997;100:907–13.
13. Ozcanli H, Coskunfirat OK, Bektas G, et al. Innervated digital artery perforator flap. J Hand Surg Am 2013;38:350–6.
14. Mitsunaga N, Mihara M, Koshima I, et al. Digital artery perforator (DAP) flaps: modifications for fingertip and finger stump reconstruction. J Plast Reconstr Aesthet Surg 2010;63:1312–7.
15. Atasoy E. Reversed cross-finger subcutaneous flap. J Hand Surg Am 1982;7:481–3.
16. Hyakusoku H, Gao JH. The "super-thin" flap. Br J Plast Surg 1994;47:457–64.
17. Regmi S, Gu JX, Zhang NC, et al. A systematic review of outcomes and complications of primary fingertip reconstruction using reverse-flow homodigital island flaps. Aesthetic Plast Surg 2016;40:277–83.
18. Lee DC, Kim JS, Ki SH, et al. Partial second toe pulp free flap for fingertip reconstruction. Plast Reconstr Surg 2008;121:899–907.
19. Lee TP, Liao CY, Wu IC, et al. Free flap from the superficial palmar branch of the radial artery (SPBRA flap) for finger reconstruction. J Trauma 2009;66:1173–9.
20. Omokawa S, Ryu J, Tang JB, et al. Vascular and neural anatomy of the thenar area of the hand: its surgical applications. Plast Reconstr Surg 1997;99:116–21.
21. Wang ZT, Zheng YM, Zhu L, et al. Exploring new frontier of microsurgery: from anatomy to clinical methods. Clin Plast Surg 2017;44:186–207.
22. Quaba AA, Davison PM. The distally-based dorsal hand flap. Br J Plast Surg 1990;43:28–39.
23. Sebastin SJ, Mendoza RT, Chong AK, et al. Application of the dorsal metacarpal artery perforator flap for resurfacing soft-tissue defects proximal to the fingertip. Plast Reconstr Surg 2011;128:166e–78e.
24. Eo S, Kim Y, Kim JY, et al. The versatility of the dorsalis pedis compound free flap in hand reconstruction. Ann Plast Surg 2008;61:157–63.
25. Hrabowski M, Kloeters O, Germann G. Reverse homodigital dorsoradial flap for thumb soft tissue reconstruction: surgical technique. J Hand Surg Am 2010;35:659–62.
26. Terán P, Carnero S, Miranda R, et al. Refinements in dorsoulnar flap of the thumb: 15 cases. J Hand Surg Am 2010;35:1356–9.

27. Elliot D, Wilson Y. V-Y advancement of the entire volar soft tissue of the thumb in distal reconstruction. J Hand Surg Br 1993;18:399–402.

28. Tang JB, Elliot D, Adani R, et al. Repair and reconstruction of thumb and finger tip injuries: a global view. Clin Plast Surg 2014;41:325–59.

29. Joshi BB. One-stage repair for distal amputation of the thumb. Plast Reconstr Surg 1970;45:613–5.

30. Büchler U, Frey HP. Retrograde posterior interosseous flap. J Hand Surg Am 1991;16:283–92.

31. Chang SM, Hou CL. The development of the distally based radial forearm flap in hand reconstruction with preservation of the radial artery. Plast Reconstr Surg 2000;106:955–97.

32. Chang SM, Hou CL, Zhang F, et al. Distally based radial forearm flap with preservation of the radial artery: anatomic, experimental, and clinical studies. Microsurgery 2003;23:328–37.

33. Ho AM, Chang J. Radial artery perforator flap. J Hand Surg 2010;35A:308–11.

34. Bertelli JA, Pagliei A. The neurocutaneous flap based on the dorsal branches of the ulnar artery and nerve: a new flap for extensive reconstructionof the hand. Plast Reconstr Surg 1998;101:1537–143.

35. Holevich-Madjarova B, Paneva-Holevich E, Topkarov V. Island flap supplied by the dorsal branch of the ulnar artery. Plast Reconstr Surg 1991;87:562–6.

36. Chen QZ, Sun YC, Chen J, et al. Comparative study of functional and aesthetically outcomes of reverse digital artery and reverse dorsal homodigital island flaps for fingertip repair. J Hand Surg Eur Vol 2015;40:935–43.

37. Sun YC, Chen QZ, Chen J, et al. Prevalence, characteristics and natural history of cold intolerance after the reverse digital artery flap. J Hand Surg Eur Vol 2016;41:171–6.

38. Lee SH, Jang JH, Kim JI, et al. Modified anterograde pedicle advancement flap in fingertip injury. J Hand Surg Eur Vol 2015;40:944–51.

39. Shen XF, Mi JY, Xue MY, et al. modified great toe wraparound flap with preservation of plantar triangular flap for reconstruction of degloving injuries of the thumb and fingers: long-term follow-up. Plast Reconstr Surg 2016;138:155–63.

40. Usami S, Kawahara S, Yamaguchi Y, et al. Homodigital artery flap reconstruction for fingertip amputation: a comparative study of the oblique triangular neurovascular advancement flap and the reverse digital artery island flap. J Hand Surg Eur Vol 2015;40:291–7.

Technical Points of 5 Free Vascularized Flaps for the Hand Repairs

Jing Chen, MD[a], Reena Bhatt, MD[b], Jin Bo Tang, MD[a],*

KEYWORDS

- Venous flap • Transverse wrist crease flap • Partial or trimmed toe transfer
- Medial plantar artery flap • Finger or thumb defect

KEY POINTS

- We present methods and key technical points of 5 less commonly used free vascularized flaps: venous flap, medial plantar artery flap, trimmed toe flap, radial artery superficial palmar branch flap from the transverse crease of the wrist, and free thenar flap.
- These 5 free flaps can solve most soft tissue defects of the digits and hand.
- The key to success of the venous flap is to eliminate the arteriovenous shunting effect of this flap.
- Partial or complete deficits of thumb or fingertips can be reconstructed by the trimmed toe flap, giving an improved appearance.
- The medial plantar artery flap provides thin and large soft tissue coverage of the hand with glabrous and nonglabrous tissue.
- The free flap from the wrist transverse crease area and the free thenar flap are based on different radial artery superficial palmar branches or their perforators. These flaps can be used for finger or thumb soft tissue defects.

INTRODUCTION

There are several methods to reconstruct soft tissue defects in the hand. Local pedicled flaps have been mainstays in treatment. However, many hand and microsurgeons are inclined to use free vascularized flap transfers in these conditions. Of particular note, radial forearm flaps have almost been entirely abandoned for hand reconstruction in China. Instead, flaps from the lower leg, such as the free anterolateral thigh (ALT) flap, are very popular. However, the ALT flap is typically quite bulky; even with skilled microsurgeons and thin patients, the super-thin ALT flap is not always reliable. The ALT flap cannot reconstruct glabrous tissue, nor can it replace the aesthetics of the fingertip.

Alternative free flaps, although less commonly used, may become first-line treatment given the ability to replace similar tissue components. These smaller free flaps are valuable in the reconstructive armamentarium of those surgeons who are well versed with microsurgical techniques.

Surgeons in different units have their own preference in flap donors. In this article, we present the experiences from Chinese microsurgeons on 5 less commonly used free vascularized flaps in hand reconstruction. In many units in China, these flaps have become the mainstays of treatment; they are routinely used for fingertip and thumb reconstruction. Their combined experience has demonstrated the reliability and versatility of these

[a] Department of Hand Surgery, Affiliated Hospital of Nantong University, 20 West Temple Road, Nantong 226001, Jiangsu, China; [b] Department of Hand and Foot Surgery, Shandong Provincial Hospital, No. 324, Jingwu Road, Jinan 250021, Shandong, China
* Corresponding author. Department of Hand Surgery, The Hand Surgery Research Center, Affiliated Hospital of Nantong University, 20 West Temple Road, Nantong 226001, Jiangsu, China.
E-mail address: jinbotang@yahoo.com

hand.theclinics.com

flaps for hand reconstruction, as well as their cosmetic value.

ARTERIALIZED VENOUS FLAP

The ideal flap should fit the functional demands of the hand while limiting donor morbidity. A venous flap potentially constitutes an ideal flap to repair a small or medium-sized defect of the hand. Although the arterialized venous flap has many advantages, it is unpopular owing to the unpredictability and published suboptimal survival rates.[1–3] We do not use this flap routinely to repair fingertip defects, but we use this flap on the volar or dorsal surface of the fingers, including the metacarpophalangeal joint region. The key to improving the survival rate of the flap is to ensure a good venous return to reduce venous congestion. Several days of altered blood flow within the flap causes an abnormal appearance of the flap for the first postoperative week; however, after a week the color of the flap will improve.

Surgical Techniques

The wounds of the injured digits are cleaned and debrided and the area of defect is measured. The artery and vein of the recipient site are dissected and tagged. In general, a dorsal digital vein and proper digital artery are the best choices. The venous flap is harvested from the palmar aspect of the ipsilateral forearm.

First, a venous tourniquet, that is, applying a tourniquet without evacuation of blood from the vessels, is applied to facilitate mapping of veins in the palmar distal or middle of the forearm (**Fig. 1**). If possible, the flap should be harvested from the ulnar aspect of the forearm. This flap

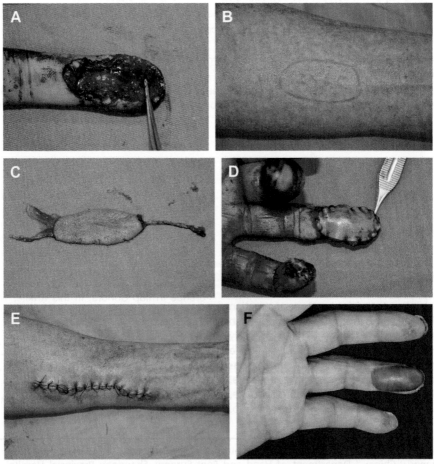

Fig. 1. Immediate venous flap transfer for a defect in the pulp of the left ring finger in a 74-year-old man. (*A*) The area of defect was 2.0 × 3.5 cm. (*B*) Three hours after injury, a venous flap was harvested from the ipsilateral volar forearm. (*C*) The flap included H-pattern veins. We performed a shunt-restricted procedure. (*D*) The flap was transferred to the recipient site and the veins of the flap were anastomosed to the digital artery and the dorsal digital vein. The appearance of the flap was pink after operation. (*E*) The donor site was sutured directly. (*F*) Appearance of the flap one and half month later. (*Courtesy of* Jing Chen, MD, Nantong, Jiangsu, China.)

can be designed to contain the medial cutaneous nerve of the forearm or palmaris longus tendon, in special circumstances.

Then, an arterial tourniquet, that is, exsanguination before applying the tourniquet, is applied to achieve a bloodless surgical field. A template of the defect is then created and transposed onto the forearm donor site in a reversed position, allowing for correct orientation of the definitive flap. An incision is made along the lateral margin of the outlined flap and carried down to the subfascial level. The flap is raised to contain skin, subcutaneous veins, and subcutaneous fat to avoid damaging the veins and subdermal plexus. Elimination of arteriovenous shunting is important. In 2007, Liu and colleagues[4] reported that they added an "opening groove," making a double-stemmed arterialized venous flap to eliminate the arteriovenous shunting effect and blood bypassing the flap to ensure sufficient "arterial" perfusion pressure. The method of making an "opening groove" is that the adipose tissue of the flaps is cut all the way up to the subdermal vascular plexus and all the communicating branches are religated while keeping the subdermal vascular network intact. Lam and colleagues[3] performed 22 shunt-restricted arterialized venous flaps for the reconstruction of digital defects and achieved 100% survival rate. The dimensions of the flaps were a mean of 2.3 × 4.5 cm^2.

In our patients, we chose H-pattern or II-pattern venous flaps and ligated the ramus communicans between the 2 main veins. In addition, we purposefully selected the smaller-caliber vein for inflow and the larger-caliber vein for outflow. We suggest the size of defects repaired by this flap should not exceed 3 × 6 cm.

Then the flap is positioned over the recipient site. The smaller vein is anastomosed to the proper digital artery and the larger-caliber vein to the dorsal digital vein. Once the anastomosis is complete, the flap will pink-up after a few minutes. The donor site is sutured directly. Close postoperative monitoring is performed. Routine postoperative anticoagulant therapy is used. After surgery, it takes a few days for the color and temperature of a venous flap to resemble those of a conventional free flap. There is swelling and venous congestion in some cases, and bleeding is common for approximately 3 or 4 days, then the appearance of the flaps gradually becomes normal.

Pros and Cons of the Venous Flaps

Pros of the flap
A major advantage is that the flap can be raised from virtually any area of the body, including the forearm, it contains subcutaneous veins, and has minimal donor site morbidity. No major artery is sacrificed. For soft tissue defects in the fingers and thumbs, this flap offers a thin and pliable flap that meets the aesthetic and functional needs of these digits. In addition, the flap can be harvested together with the palmaris longus tendon or cutaneous sensory nerve when necessary. The flap size is also flexible; it can cover the proximal half of the digits or a reasonably sized area in the palm.

Cons of the flap
A disadvantage is the unpredictable survival. However, more recently, several groups have reported use of this flap in hand reconstruction and found that it has a predictably high survival rate and optimal soft tissue coverage with appropriate ligation of the communicating vessels.[4–7] In China, a few centers regularly use this flap; the reported survival rates are 77% to 96%.[4–7] We also use this flap for small to medium-sized defects of the fingers, but would caution against reconstruction of a larger defect.

TRANSVERSE WRIST CREASE FLAP (FREE RADIAL ARTERY SUPERFICIAL PALMAR BRANCH FLAP OF THE WRIST)

A transverse free radial artery superficial palmar branch (RASPB) flap can be harvested from the flexor aspect of the wrist.[8,9] In China, this flap is popularly called the "transverse wrist crease flap," as this flap is harvested from the area of the proximal transverse wrist crease. Such terminology makes this flap distinctive from the free thenar flap, which is based on other RASPBs. The transverse wrist crease flap is attractive because it is a very thin flap and the donor site can be closed directly.

In our experience, the dissection of the transverse wrist crease flap is easier than that of the free thenar flap. Cosmetically, its donor site is less obvious, as the incision for flap harvest overlaps or parallels the proximal transverse wrist crease.

Surgical Techniques

The RASPB usually divides from the radial artery 1 or 2 cm proximal to the distal wrist crease; the diameter is 0.8 to 3.5 mm.[8] There are 2 to 5 branches on the flexor aspect of the wrist region and these perforators lie on the side of the palmaris longus tendon.[8,9] The artery is usually accompanied by 1 or 2 venae comitantes. On the proximal side of the forearm, 1 or 2 subcutaneous veins of adequate size and length are chosen for flap drainage. The sensory innervation of this flap is the medial antebrachial cutaneous nerve or palmar cutaneous branch of the median nerve.

If possible, the origin, perforators, and the path of the RASPB are detected and marked preoperatively with Doppler ultrasound. Using a brachial plexus block, a tourniquet is used to achieve a bloodless surgical field. The wound is debrided, and the area of defect is measured. The artery and vein of the recipient site are dissected and marked. The flap is tailored according to the shape of the wound. The size of the flap is designed as 110% to 120% of the defect area.

First, the radial margin of the flap is incised and the origin of the RASPB is dissected. Then the incision is made at the proximal margin of the outlined flap and a sufficient length of superficial volar veins is dissected proximally and transected. The

dissection is carried down to the subfascial level (**Fig. 2**). The RASPB is dissected from the ulnar to the radial side and distally under the deep fascia until reaching the origin of the RASPB. During flap dissection, the cutaneous perforating branches of the RASPB may not be visible. However, there are typically at least 2 cutaneous perforators in this flap.

The tourniquet is temporarily released to check the circulation of the flap. Once confirmed, the flap pedicle is divided. The flap is positioned over the recipient site. The artery of the flap is anastomosed to the proper digital artery and the superficial palmar or volar veins are connected with the dorsal digital veins. Neurorrhaphy may be performed between the median palmar cutaneous branch and the digital nerves. The donor site is closed directly. Chi and colleagues[10] introduced

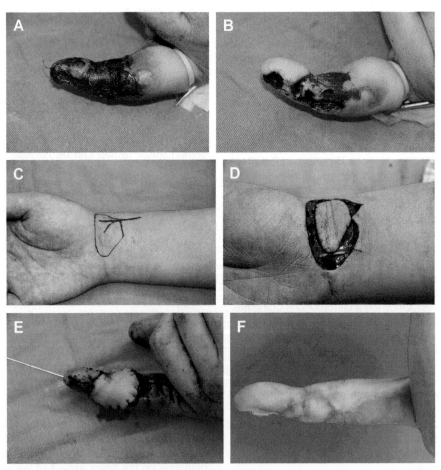

Fig. 2. The transverse wrist crease flap was applied in a 32-year-old woman. (*A*) The skin of the index finger had partial necrosis. (*B*) The defect area was 2.5 × 3.5 cm with tendon exposure. (*C*) The flap was designed and harvested from the flexor aspect of the ipsilateral wrist. (*D*) The circulation was excellent after temporary release of the tourniquet. (*E*) The flap was transferred to the recipient site and the artery and veins of the flap were anastomosed to the digital artery and the dorsal digital vein. The perfusion of the flap was robust. (*F*) Appearance of the transferred flap 4 months later. (*Courtesy of* Jing Chen, MD, Nantong, Jiangsu, China.)

a modified technique: a bilobed innervated RASPB flap. At least 2 cutaneous perforators were identified. The 2 flaps based on a common vascular pedicle were designed on the basis of the 2 cutaneous perforators. This technique was applied successfully in 12 patients of degloving injuries of the digits.

Pros and Cons of This Flap

Pros of the flap

The harvesting and transfer of the flap is performed on the same upper limb. No major artery is sacrificed. The flap can be used as a vascularized tendon or nerve graft when it involves a palmaris longus tendon or the palmar cutaneous branch of the median nerve. Glabrous tissue is available for reconstruction of volar digital defects.

Cons of the flap

The length of the arterial pedicle of this flap is relatively short. Sensory loss in the thenar area occurs when the palmar cutaneous branch of the median nerve is harvested. The flap is only suitable for small to moderate-size defects of the hand and fingers.

We use this flap to repair defects of the pulp or the volar aspect of digits because of the ideal thickness and texture of this flap. We think that the dissection and exposure of the pedicle is the key to success. We often find that the branches of the RASPB are intertwined with the veins and dissection should be careful. In addition, there is a limit to the length of the pedicle.[8–10]

PARTIAL OR TRIMMED TOE TRANSFER

The nail, pulp, and paronychia all play unique roles and are challenging to reproduce aesthetically. The trimmed toe flap can replace like with like for partial or complete deficits of fingertips, such as partial nail and pulp defects or more complex injuries. When the composite tissue flap is harvested from the great toe, that is, a *paronychial-pulp-nailbed-bone flap*, for thumb reconstruction, the lateral aspect of the great toe is favorable as a donor, given shoe wear and weight bearing.[11–19]

Surgical Techniques

A thin osteo-onychocutaneous flap can be raised from the lateral (fibular) side of the great toe for composite loss of skin, nail, and bone from the thumb (**Fig. 3**).

After debridement, the defect to be reconstructed was measured. The flap was designed on the ipsilateral great toe; however, if the region to reconstruct is the radial thumb, then the contralateral great toe is ideal. For small partial fingertip

reconstructions that are not the thumb, the medial (tibial) side of the second toe can be harvested; ipsilateral or contralateral as needed. The partial great toe graft can be used for fingertip reconstruction.

The pedicle artery is the first dorsal or plantar metatarsal artery, the lateral plantar or dorsal digital artery of the great toe, or the medial plantar or dorsal digital artery of the second toe, depending on the flap harvested. The vein is traditionally the dorsal digital vein of the selected toe or the dorsal metatarsal vein. The plantar digital nerve can be harvested; in addition, branches of the deep peroneal nerve to the dorsum of the toe can be used. Other designs of partial toe transfers or flaps are illustrated in **Figs. 4** and **5**.

A preoperative angiogram is not routinely performed, but should be considered if there is a relative risk of peripheral vascular disease. Other indicators for further vascular assessment include patients older than 50 years or those with diabetes, tobacco abuse, or history of cardiovascular disease.[15]

Pros and Cons of This Flap

The benefits of these microvascular flaps from the toe are replacing like with like and the flexibility of flap design. Downsides include the small caliber of the vessels, especially the digital vessels, the variability in the anatomy, nail notching, and donor site morbidity.[18,19]

MEDIAL PLANTAR ARTERY FLAP

Extensive soft tissue loss with exposed tendon or bone in the hand can be addressed by pedicled or free flaps depending on the location, degree, and type of trauma and size and functional needs of the region of interest. Challenges inherent to the hand include the difficulty of replacing glabrous skin and the desire and often necessity for sensation. The medial plantar flap can address many of these needs and can be combined with the medialis pedis flap to replace nonglabrous and glabrous regions in one flap.

In the setting of acute injury, with loss of perfusion to the fingertip secondary to volar injury with combined neurovascular injury, the fasciocutaneous free medial plantar artery with sensory nerve can allow for primary reconstruction with revascularization of the finger. Combined flaps of medialis pedis and medial plantar (instep) flaps are a good combination, as the pedicles of the 2 flaps are branches of the common medial plantar artery.[20]

The lateral or superficial branch of the medial plantar artery provides perforating cutaneous branches between the abductor hallucis and the plantar fascia, the main artery to the medial plantar

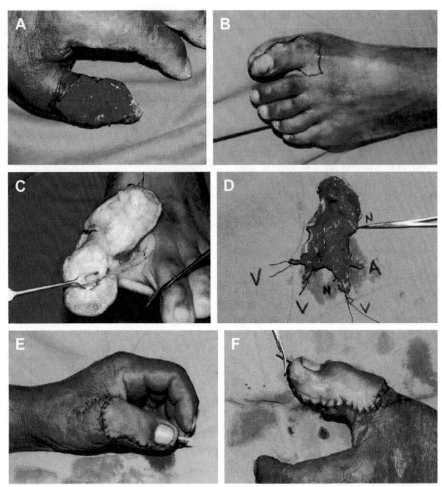

Fig. 3. (*A*) A patient with composite soft tissue loss of the dorsal left thumb. (*B*) A partial great toe flap has been planned, including nail, tuft for bony support of the distal nail, and fibular hyponychium. (*C*) A small region of tuft of the distal phalanx was removed en bloc with the flap. (*D*) The undersurface of the flap is seen with veins (v), artery (A), and sensory nerves (N) labeled. (*E*) The flap was inset to the prepared thumb recipient site after open reduction internal fixation with 1 Kirschner wire (K-wire) together with anastomoses of 1 artery (ulnar digital artery), 2 veins (dorsal veins), and repair of the nerve in the donor to the ulnar proper digital nerve and another to the radial sensory branch of the thumb. (*F*) Lateral view of the repaired thumb after transfer. (*Courtesy of* Chao Chen, MD, Jinan, Shandong, China.)

artery flap. The midline or axis of the flap is over the septum between the abductor hallucis and flexor digitorum brevis for the medial plantar artery instep flap alone versus over the medial axis centered on the navicular tubercle, if the medialis pedis flap is used. Important anatomic markers include the posterior tibial artery transitioning to the medial plantar artery (MPA) past the tarsal tunnel, under the abductor hallucis muscle. The artery continues within the septum between the abductor hallucis and flexor digitorum brevis; at the level of the talo-navicular joint, the MPA divides into deep and superficial branches. Perforating branches of the deep branch of the MPA vascularize the medialis pedis, whereas the superficial branch of the

MPA provides blood flow to the medial plantar or instep flap. The superficial branch passes within the intermuscular septum between the abductor hallucis and the flexor digitorum brevis, whereas the deep branch remains deep, parallel, and under the abductor hallucis along the medial aspect.[21]

The medial plantar nerve passes between the abductor hallucis and the flexor hallucis brevis muscles. After providing innervation to the flexor hallucis brevis, it continues on as the medial digital nerve to the great toe; this nerve can provide sensory innervation to the flap. The veins for the flap are the dorsal veins at the instep, branches contributing to the saphenous system, as well as the venae comitantes of the respective arteries.

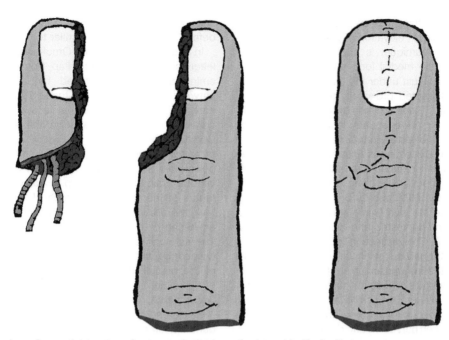

Fig. 4. Design of a partial toe transfer to repair the loss of a lateral half of a finger.

Surgical Techniques

The recipient site defect is outlined after adequate debridement. The recipient artery, veins, and nerve are prepared. The planned flap is designed over the instep of the foot in the non–weight-bearing region and can be extended medially and proximally for the combined medialis pedis-medial plantar flap. Using compression of the saphenous vein, any medial veins, at the medial

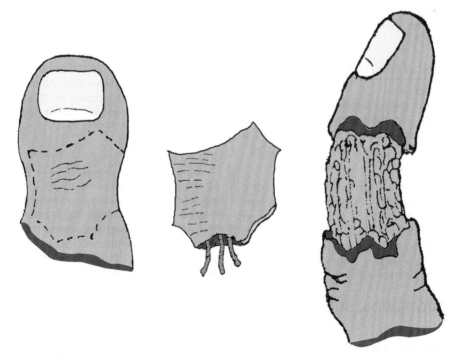

Fig. 5. Design of a flap from the toe to cover a finger soft tissue defect.

aspect of the flap, that engorge are marked out before tourniquet elevation (**Fig. 6**).

After the tourniquet is applied, an incision is made over the medial foot, the cutaneous veins are superficial just under the skin and need to be carefully dissected proximally to gain an appropriate length. These are then divided proximally after obtaining an adequate length; 2 veins are harvested. The venae comitantes of the artery are often used. Dissection is usually medial to lateral and distal to proximal. The abductor hallucis is retracted laterally exposing the deep (medial) branch of the MPA and its branches. Perforating branches to the skin with the medial branch are included and harvested and dissected proximally to the MPA. The dissection is then carried over the abductor hallucis, which is retracted medially, exposing the intermuscular septum between the abductor hallucis and flexor digitorum brevis. The superficial or lateral branch of the MPA, with perforating cutaneous branches and intermuscular septum, is then harvested and dissected proximally to the MPA. At the distal forefoot aspect of the flap, the medial digital nerve is identified, divided, and retained with the flap if needed. The abductor hallucis often requires division at its origin to adequately expose the MPA and posterior tibial artery.

Next, the flap is divided at the MPA, and transferred to the recipient site. The abductor hallucis is repaired if divided during the procedure; the wound is reconstructed with a full-thickness skin graft. An overlying bolster, pressure dressing, or negative-pressure dressing and splint are applied to donor site. The upper extremity injury is immobilized as well.[22–24]

Pros and Cons of This Flap

Pros of the flap
Glabrous and nonglabrous options are available in many variations. The glabrous skin on the palms is durable and assists in prehensile function. The flap can be sensate.

Cons of the flap
The length of the MPA can be short, 2 to 3 cm; thus, the posterior tibial artery may require harvesting as well. There can be anatomic variations in the arterial supply of the flap. Additionally, a skin graft is required for flaps larger than 2 to 3 cm. Non–weight-bearing status is required until adequate skin graft healing.[25]

FREE FASCIOCUTANEOUS SENSATE THENAR FLAP

The free thenar flap is a good choice in patients who have no desire to use their foot as a donor site and have a small to moderate-sized volar defect. It provides tissue similar to finger pulp.

In cadaveric studies, Omokawa and colleagues[26] found that the flap from the thenar eminence was vascularized by a cutaneous network to the skin from the thenar RASPB, which emerges 1 to 2 cm proximal to the distal wrist crease along the ulnar aspect of the radial artery. Constant skin territories of 3×4 cm over the proximal abductor pollicis brevis and opponens pollicis are supplied by this arterial branch. The venous drainage of this flap is the venae comitantes of the superficial branch of the radial artery, the dorsal veins emanating from the thenar eminence or the superficial volar forearm veins. The sensory territory to the thenar eminence is divided between the palmar cutaneous branch of the median nerve and the sensory branches of the radial nerve and lateral antebrachial cutaneous nerve.

Sassu and colleagues[27] described an independent branch of the radial artery that, when available, is the preferable pedicle to the free thenar flap. They described an independent branch of the radial artery, which emerges 2 to 3 cm proximal to the wrist crease. This artery is slightly narrower than the superficial branch, making it an ideal size match for the digital artery at the recipient site. This vessel was present in 7 of 14 patients.

There is a concentration of perforators around the scaphoid tubercle area; this should be a standard landmark for free thenar flaps. This flap also can be designed on small perforating vessels from the superficial palmar arch or superficial branch of the radial artery with many variations of flap configuration, but the pedicle is short and requires a difficult dissection. Additionally, Akita and colleagues[28] reported on 8 patients with perforator-based pedicled thenar flaps for digital defects.

Surgical Techniques

After appropriate debridement and preparation of the recipient site vessels and nerve, a template is created. The free thenar flap is marked (**Fig. 7**). The perforator-based free thenar flap can have many variations in design. The superficial branch of the radial artery can be felt over the scaphoid tubercle. Doppler is useful to trace the course of the radial artery and perforators about the scaphoid tubercle within the thenar eminence. Using manual compression proximal to the region of interest, or gravity, engorgement of superficial dorsal or volar veins emanating from the thenar region can be marked out. As described previously, the radial

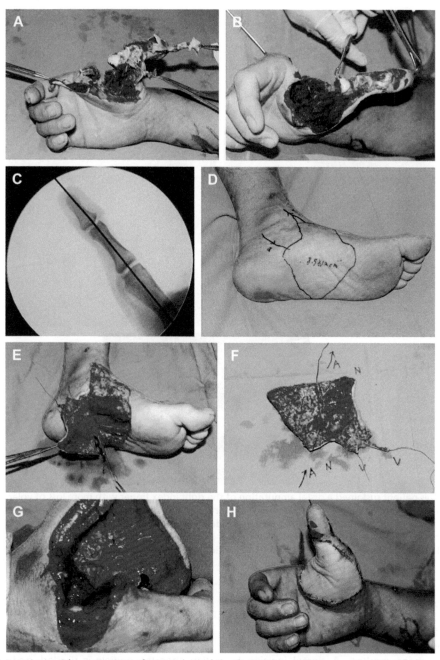

Fig. 6. (*A*) A patient with composite soft tissue loss of the first webspace, ulnar, and volar right thumb. (*B*) The wound has been debrided and irrigated aggressively. (*C*) A single longitudinal K-wire has been used to stabilize the 2 thumb joints. (*D*) Given the lack of perfusion to the thumb, acute reconstruction ensued. An MPA for glabrous tissue was designed and extended proximally over the region of the medialis pedis flap for nonglabrous reconstruction. (*E*) The flap was raised based on the medial plantar artery in flow-through fashion to reestablish the flow to the thumb tip. (*F*) The undersurface of the flap with 1 artery that is flow-through, 2 veins, and sensory cutaneous nerve is demonstrated. (*G*) The flap is inset in flow-through fashion to reconstruct the ulnar digital artery, with glabrous tissue replacing the glabrous skin loss of the thumb and palm. The glabrous portion of the instep was oriented volarly, whereas the nonglabrous supple medialis pedis skin was oriented dorsally. The superficial branch of the MPA was inset to the defect of the ulnar digital artery to provide vascularization to the flap as well as flow-through to the thumb tip. The superficial veins of the flap were anastomosed to the dorsal veins of the hand. The hallucal medial digital nerve was inset to the nerve defect of the ulnar digital nerve. The flexor pollicis longus will be reconstructed at a later date. (*H*) Final inset of the flap is shown. (*Courtesy of Chao Chen, MD, Jinan, Shandong, China.*)

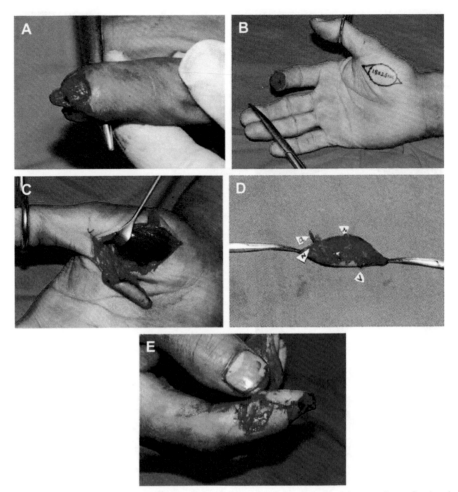

Fig. 7. (*A*) This patient sustained a distal amputation of the right index finger with more loss of volar than dorsal tissue. There was exposed bone with maintenance of more than half of the sterile matrix. (*B*) To preserve length, a sensate fasciocutaneous perforator thenar free flap is designed immediately after debridement. (*C*) Flap elevation. (*D*) The undersurface of the flap with 1 artery (A), 2 veins (V), and sensory cutaneous nerve (N) is demonstrated. (*E*) Inset of the flap is illustrated with visualization of 1 venous anastomosis. (*Courtesy of* Li Wen Hao, MD, Jinan, Shandong, China.)

artery superficial branch usually branches 1 to 2 cm proximal to the wrist crease.

The perforator-based free flap should be based on the courses of Doppler-detected perforators, which have been marked. A dorsal incision is made; the dorsal veins are dissected and divided and maintained with the flap. A superficial branch of the radial sensory nerve or lateral antebrachial sensory nerve can be included, during the radial dissection at the proximal aspect of the flap elevation and included with the flap. Dissection is carried down to the thenar muscular fascia, which is included with the flap and elevated ulnarly. The cutaneous perforators are identified and traced proximally, distally, or dorsally, and even intramuscularly. Proximal superficial veins can be identified as well, and included with the flap. Once the pedicle length is adequate (ranging from 1 to 2 cm), the flap is elevated but maintained on the perforating vessels. The tourniquet is deflated to demonstrate good perfusion to the flap, then the pedicle is divided, and transferred to the recipient site. The donor site is closed primarily.

Modifications of the flap have been described. Iwuagwu and colleagues[29] transposed the flap to the midpalmar crease, basing the flap on the deep branch of the volar branch of the radial artery with better cosmesis of the donor site, similar to a carpal tunnel release incision. In 14 patients undergoing free thenar flaps of an average size of 4.6 × 2.4 cm, Sassu and colleagues[27] reported 2 reexplorations, 1 for arterial and 1 for venous thrombosis, with successful salvage.

Pros and Cons of This Flap

Pros of this flap

The free thenar flap with sensory innervation sacrifices only a nondominant artery, it replaces glabrous tissue, and there is good vessel-size match for the digital vessels, the opportunity for some sensory recovery, and all the surgery is performed on the same limb.

Cons of this flap

This flap may lead to neuroma formation, injury to the recurrent motor branch of the median nerve, and a widened scar. The dissection can be tedious if perforator based. There is a limit to the size of the flap, that is, less than 1.5 to 2.0-cm width for primary closure. If the radial artery superficial branch is used, vascular reconstruction may be required if that is the dominant artery to the superficial arch, the vessels may be very small, and the anatomy may be aberrant, especially if perforator based.[30] This flap is technically more challenging and its drawbacks appear greater than the transverse wrist crease flap described earlier.

SUMMARY

Soft tissue defects with exposed tendon or bone in the hand can be repaired with pedicled flaps. However, free vascularized flaps offer a few distinct advantages and can be the ideal choice under certain circumstances. Some surgeons prefer free vascularized flaps in repairing defects of the hand because of versatile donor selection and repair of like with like tissue. The described 5 free vascularized flaps reconstruct complex soft tissue losses of the hand without harvesting major arteries and can improve the cosmetic appearance. They augment function and can be quite reliable in hand repairs with appropriate planning and microsurgical expertise. Additionally, modification of the venous flap can optimize the survival rate and thus encourage greater interest in free flap use in hand surgery. The MPA flap can be combined with the medialis pedis flap to resurface large defects in nonglabrous and glabrous regions of the hand. The free transverse wrist crease flap and free thenar flap are good choices in patients who do not want surgery on their foot but have a small to moderate-sized volar defect. They provide tissue similar to the finger pulp.

ACKNOWLEDGMENTS

Dr Reena Bhatt gives her special thanks to Dr Chao Chen and Dr Lin Feng Liu in the Hand and Foot Surgical Center, Shandong Provincial Hospital, for including operative pictures of their cases. She is currently an assistant professor of plastic surgery, The Warren Alpert Medical School of Brown University, Providence, Rhode Island. Gratitude was extended to Dr Zeng Tao Wang and his team, Dr Shen Qiang Qiu, Dr Li Shan Zang, Dr Li Wen Hao, Dr Chao Xi Wen, Dr Yun Peng Wang, Dr Di Zhang, Dr Lan Wei Xu, Dr Xiao Bin Chen, Dr Wei Kou, and Dr Gang Chen.

REFERENCES

1. Chen HC, Tang YB, Noordhoff MS. Four types of venous flaps for wound coverage: a clinical appraisal. J Trauma 1991;31:1286–93.
2. Yan H, Brooks D, Ladner R, et al. Arterialized venous flaps: a review of the literature. Microsurgery 2010; 30:472–8.
3. Lam WL, Lin WN, Bell D, et al. The physiology, microcirculation and clinical application of the shunt-restricted arterialized venous flaps for the reconstruction of digital defects. J Hand Surg Eur Vol 2013;38:352–65.
4. Liu XG, Zhang MS, Yang JG, et al. Application of modified arterialized venous flap. Chin J Hand Surg 2007;23:224–6.
5. Lin YT, Henry SL, Lin CH, et al. The shunt-restricted arterialized venous flap for hand/digit reconstruction: enhanced perfusion, decreased congestion, and improved reliability. J Trauma 2010;69:399–404.
6. Pittet B, Quinodoz P, Alizadeh N, et al. Optimizing the arterialized venous flap. Plast Reconstr Surg 2008;122:1681–9.
7. Xu YF, Wu MY, Zhang YF, et al. The application of improved arterialized venous flaps in the defects of fingers. Chin J Microsurg 2011;34:321–2.
8. Sakai S. Free flap from the flexor aspect of the wrist for resurfacing defects of the hand and fingers. Plast Reconstr Surg 2003;111:1412–20.
9. Wang ZT, Zheng YM, Zhu L, et al. Exploring new frontiers of microsurgery: from anatomy to clinical methods. Clin Plast Surg 2017;44:211–31.
10. Chi ZL, Yang P, Song D, et al. Reconstruction of totally degloved fingers: a novel application of the bilobed spiraled innervated radial artery superficial palmar branch perforator flap design provides for primary donor-site closure. Surg Radiol Anat 2017; 39:547–57.
11. Wenhai S, Chen C, Wang Z, et al. Full-length finger reconstruction for proximal amputation with expanded wraparound great toe flap and vascularized second toe joint. Ann Plast Surg 2016;77: 539–46.
12. Tsai T, D'Agostino L, Fang Y, et al. Compound flap from the great toe and vascularized joints from the second toe for posttraumatic thumb reconstruction

at the level of the proximal metacarpal bone. Micro-surgery 2009;29:179–83.

13. Hou Z, Zou J, Wang Z, et al. Anatomical classification of the first dorsal metatarsal artery and its clinical application. Plast Reconstr Surg 2013;132: 1028e–39e.

14. Koshima I, Kawada S, Etoh H, et al. Free combined thin wrap-around flap with a second toe proximal interphalangeal joint transfer for reconstruction of the thumb. Plast Reconstr Surg 1995;96:1205–10.

15. Woo S, Lee G, Kim K, et al. Immediate partial great toe transfer for the reconstruction of composite defects of the distal thumb. Plast Reconstr Surg 2006;117:1906–15.

16. Tomaino M. Donor site toe morbidity should not be underestimated when considering options for thumb reconstruction. J Hand Surg Br 2000;25:228–9.

17. Lin P, Sebastin S, Ono S, et al. A systematic review of outcomes of toe-to-thumb transfers for isolated traumatic thumb amputation. Hand 2011;6:235–43.

18. Tang JB, Elliot D, Adani R, et al. Repair and reconstruction of thumb and finger tip injuries: a global view. Clin Plast Surg 2014;41:325–59.

19. Nikkhah D, Martin N, Pickford M. Paediatric toe-to-hand transfer: an assessment of outcomes from a single unit. J Hand Surg Eur Vol 2016;41:281–94.

20. Chen C, Hao L, Sun W, et al. Glabrous flow-through flaps for simultaneous resurfacing, revascularization, and reinnervation of digits. Ann Plast Surg 2016;77:547–54.

21. Rodriguez-Vega M. Medialis pedis flap in the reconstruction of palmar skin defects of the digits: clarifying the anatomy of the medial plantar artery. Ann Plast Surg 2014;72:542–52.

22. Chai Y, Wang C, Wen G, et al. Combined medialis pedis and medial plantar fasciocutaneous flaps based on the medial plantar pedicle for reconstruction of complex soft tissue defects in the hand. Microsurgery 2011;31:45–50.

23. Okada M, Saito H, Kazuki K, et al. Combined medialis pedis and medial plantar fasciocutaneous flaps for coverage of soft tissue defects of multiple adjacent fingers. Microsurgery 2014;34:454–8.

24. Kim S, Hong J, Chung Y, et al. Sensate sole-to-sole reconstruction using the combined medial plantar and medialis pedis free flap. Ann Plast Surg 2001; 47:461–4.

25. Oh S, Koh S, Chung C. Twin digital and in-step neurovascularised free flaps for reconstruction of the degloved mutilated hands. J Plast Reconstr Aesthet Surg 2010;63:1853–9.

26. Omokawa S, Ryu J, Tang J, et al. Vascular and neural anatomy of the thenar area of the hand: its surgical applications. Plast Reconstr Surg 1997;99: 116–21.

27. Sassu P, Lin C, Lin Y, et al. Fourteen cases of free thenar flap. A rare indication in digital reconstruction. Ann Plast Surg 2008;60:260–6.

28. Akita S, Kuroki T, Yoshimoto S, et al. Reconstruction of a fingertip with a thenar perforator island flap. J Plast Surg Hand Surg 2011;45:294–9.

29. Iwuagwu FC, Orkar SK, Siddiqui A. Reconstruction of volar skin and soft tissue defects of the digits including the pulp: experience with the free SUPBRA flap. J Plast Reconstr Aesthet Surg 2015;68: 26–34.

30. Yan H, Fan C, Gao W, et al. Finger pulp reconstruction with free flaps from the upper extremity. Microsurgery 2012;32:406–14.

Strong Digital Flexor Tendon Repair, Extension-Flexion Test, and Early Active Flexion: Experience in 300 Tendons

Jin Bo Tang, MD[a],*, Xiang Zhou, MD[b], Zhang Jun Pan, MD[c], Jun Qing, MD[b], Ke Tong Gong, MD[d], Jing Chen, MD[a]

KEYWORDS

- Flexor tendon • Multistrand repair • Digital extension-flexion test • Early active motion

KEY POINTS

- The mainstays of Asian practice in primary tendon repair are a strong core tendon repair with sufficient venting of the critical pulleys, followed by a combined passive and active exercise program incorporating early active digital flexion.
- We are moving toward freer early motion, without protection from a splint during exercises.
- Interim clinical data indicate that slight or modest bulkiness of the repair site is not harmful to outcomes, although marked bulkiness should always be avoided. Such bulkiness appears unavoidable, because the core repair has to be tensioned to resist gapping.
- A slightly lengthy venting in the sheath and pulley is preferred by some surgeons to allow tendon motion; these surgeons have not observed adverse effects on hand function.
- The digital extension-flexion test has become routine and is an important step in checking the quality of the repair during surgery.

INTRODUCTION

Over the past 2 decades, repair and rehabilitation methods of primary repair of the digital flexor tendon have changed. Key techniques developed over this period include strong tendon repair methods (typically multistrand), venting of the critical pulleys, an intraoperative digital extension-flexion test of repair quality, and early postoperative active motion.[1–5] Improvements in repair outcomes have been demonstrated by hand centers with a history of tendon-related research.[6–8] However, improved outcomes are limited to teams with established reputations or track records in hand tendon repair. In addition, the number of repairs reported is usually not large and reports often do not incorporate all the critical techniques.

In this article, we outline the interim results from ongoing investigations in several units. Surgeons in these units now perform digital flexor tendon repairs according to a treatment protocol. Before they adopted the protocol, they had no history of tendon-related research; they had not used any of the repair and rehabilitation methods described in the protocol. The surgeons involved are junior or

[a] Department of Hand Surgery, The Hand Surgery Research Center, Affiliated Hospital of Nantong University, Nantong, Jiangsu, China; [b] Department of Surgery, Jiangyin People's Hospital, Jiangyin, Jiangsu, China; [c] Department of Surgery, Yixing People's Hospital, Yixing, Jiangsu, China; [d] Department of Hand Surgery, Tianjing Hospital, Tianjing, China
* Corresponding author. Department of Hand Surgery, The Hand Surgery Research Center, Affiliated Hospital of Nantong University, 20 West Temple Road, Nantong 226001, Jiangsu, China.
E-mail address: jinbotang@yahoo.com

Hand Clin 33 (2017) 455–463
http://dx.doi.org/10.1016/j.hcl.2017.04.012
0749-0712/17/© 2017 Elsevier Inc. All rights reserved.

midlevel attending surgeons. At the end of this article we outline current practice of digital flexor tendon repair in Asian countries.

CLINICAL METHODS AND PROTOCOL

Four years ago, the lead author (JBT) formulated a protocol that is a simple list of techniques and principles to guide the repair of a digital flexor tendon. This protocol is translated into English as follows.

Indications and Inclusion of Patients

The protocol is used for any zone 1 to 3 acute digital flexor tendon injury, whether clean cut or with severe soft tissue injury, requiring direct repair, without a lengthy tendon defect.

Operative Methods

Tendons should ideally be repaired on the day of injury; if not on that day, certainly within 1 or 2 weeks of injury with temporary skin closure on the day of injury. A Bruner zig-zag incision is made to expose the tendons. The flexor digitorum profundus (FDP) tendon or flexor pollicis longus (FPL) tendon is repaired with an M-Tang repair (6-strand) (**Fig. 1**) as the core suture using 4-0 looped sutures (Holycon, Nantong, Jiangsu,

China).[1,5] In some cases, at the surgeon's discretion, a U-shaped Tang repair (4-strand) can be used instead. A 5-0 or 6-0 suture is used to make a simple running peripheral suture. The key points in performing a core tendon suture are (1) to ensure 0.7 to 1 cm purchase in both tendon stumps, as too short a purchase decreases repair strength; and (2) to keep tension across the core suture, avoiding a loose suture repair. Some bulkiness in the repair site is common and typically presents no major problem. In repairing an FDP tendon close to the A2 pulley, the pulley should be vented through its midline over one-half or two-thirds of its length. When the tendon is cut close to the A4 pulley, the pulley may need to be vented completely (**Fig. 2**). It is important is to identify the A2 and A4 pulleys correctly during surgery. All surgeons who adopt this protocol should consult relevant publications to master the locations and lengths of both pulleys. The other annular pulleys should be retained as often as possible, but may be vented if required to enhance tendon gliding. The overall length of pulley-sheath venting should not exceed 2 cm. The flexor digitorum superficialis (FDS) tendon may be left unrepaired if the surgeon finds it overly difficult (or the surgeon may not repair the FDSs in all cases, which is also acceptable).

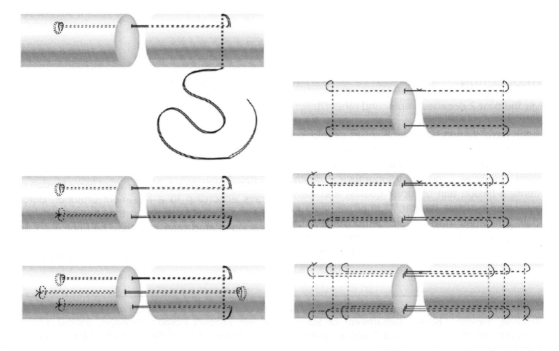

M-Tang repair (6-strand)   Asymmetric triple Kessler repair (6-strand)

Fig. 1. Methods of making a strong tendon repair are on the left: M-Tang method; U-Tang method is a 4-strand repair (shown in the middle), which omits 2 strands of the M-Tang repair. Right: The asymmetric triple Kessler method was listed in the protocol as a backup for the occasion when looped sutures are unavailable.

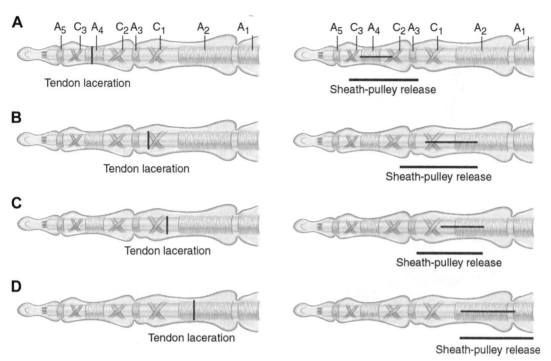

Fig. 2. On the right column under each drawing of the finger, the red lines directly over the pulleys show the original proposal of the lengths of the pulley venting; the lengths of pulley-venting in real-world practice of surgeons in 3 units are shown in dark red. The corresponding tendon cut sites are shown on the left column.

Digital Extension-Flexion Test During Surgery

This test is performed immediately after completion of the tendon repair to check quality of the repair. The test consists of 3 parts (**Fig. 3**): passive full extension of the digit to ensure the tendon repair site shows no gapping; then passive flexion of the digit to confirm that gliding is smooth; and finally pushing the digit to almost full flexion to check whether the tendon repair site (usually a bit bulky) impinges against the edge of the sheath or a pulley. If the repair is loose, the repair site will gap; such a repair should be strengthened with the addition of a tighter 2-strand or 4-strand repair. If the repair site is catching on the sheath or pulley edges, the pulley or sheath should be vented further, until smooth, unrestricted motion of the repair site is confirmed.

After surgery, a short dorsal forearm splint is applied with the wrist in neutral or a slightly flexed position, and the metacarpophalangeal (MP) joint in a moderately flexed position. The splint should be straight beyond the MP joint and should extend past the finger or thumb tip. The wrist position for splinting is not important, but should avoid marked wrist flexion (which will be uncomfortable) or marked extension (which will add unnecessary tension to the repaired tendon).

Full Range of Passive Digital Motion with Early Active Flexion After Surgery

Motion exercises should start 3 or 4 days after surgery, which is usually the time of the first dressing change. Exercise sessions should occur every 2 hours during both daytime and evening. Out-of-splint digital motion is encouraged in each session; multiple passive motion is performed first, followed by active digital flexion and extension no fewer than 30 to 40 times. However, in the first 3 to 4 weeks, only partial active digital flexion is allowed, which can be performed with or without the splint, but during the intervals between exercises and at night, the hand should be protected with a splint. Starting in weeks 4 or 5, a full range of active flexion is allowed; the splint is discarded after week 6. Active use of the hand is allowed over the next 3 weeks, but not against resistance. Passive digital flexion and extension over the full range of motion is stressed from week 1 to 6, which is key to decreasing joint stiffness. Therapy continues as long as necessary.

PRACTICE AND VARIATIONS AMONG 3 HAND-REPAIR UNITS

The previously described protocol was given to the surgeons in 3 units in 3 different cities, along with recent literature to update the surgeons' knowledge

A

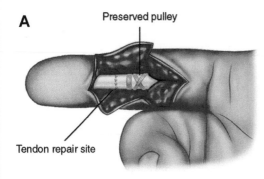

Preserved pulley

Tendon repair site

B   Finger moderately flexed

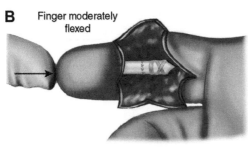

C   Finger markedly flexed

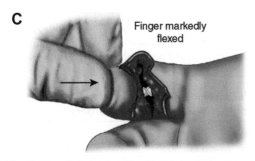

Fig. 3. The digital extension-flexion test has 3 parts: (A) full extension; (B) moving from full extension to moderate flexion; and (C) moving toward full flexion.

and, importantly, to help them understand the protocol and its key techniques. They were also offered a book in Chinese (published by the lead author) containing detailed explanations in plain Chinese of why and how a repair should be performed.[9] In addition, the surgeons were given a video of a 6-strand repair for training purposes.

The surgeons took intraoperative photographs and videos of selected patients to allow the lead author to assess technical variations among the surgeons in their use of the protocol as well as to make detailed assessments of the methods of these surgeons, which might differ from those of the lead author. The following are some noteworthy variations in their real-world practice, as noted from the intraoperative and postoperative photographs and videos:

1. Repair sites are usually much bulkier or less even compared with the lead author's usual practice
2. The pulley and sheath venting is in some cases much longer than what the lead author usually allows (**Fig. 2**); the lead author usually vents through a confined area
3. Out-of-splint motion exercise is common

Except for a small percentage (<5%) of patients who could not be called back for examinations after 6 months, photographs were taken of all patients during follow-up, showing maximal digital flexion and extension. Photographs were reviewed by a surgeon on the team and an additional independent reviewer (who is a hand surgeon but not in any of the 3 units assessed). **Table 1** summarizes the patient data and the distribution of repairs in the digits. Because of the large number of patients involved and because the investigation is ongoing,

Table 1
The numbers of digits of flexor tendons treated in Jiangyin Hospital (January 2014–April 2017), Yixing Hospital (January 2014–February 2017), and Tianjing Hospital (August 2016–May 2017) according to the protocol

Digits and Zones	Jiangyin Hospital	Yixing Hospital	Tianjing Hospital
Fingers, flexor digitorum profundus tendons			
Zone 1	11	10	6
Zone 2	116	83	7
Zone 3	14	9	0
Total	141 (114 patients)	102 (67 patients)	13 (8 patients)
Thumbs, flexor pollicis longus tendons			
Zone 1	2	3	0
Zone 2	16	14	2
Zone 3	5	2	0
Total	23 (23 patients)	19 (19 patients)	2 (2 patients)
Total digits	164 (137 patients)	121 (86 patients)	15 (10 patients)

only finger repairs in zone 2 were reviewed in detail. The excellent or good outcomes in the 3 units were 83%, 87%, and 86% based on follow-up of the first sets of consecutive sets of patients with flexor tendon cuts in the fingers (54, 60, and 7 fingers, respectively) according to the Strickland criteria. Only 1 rupture occurred, in a finger of a male worker who regained full use of his hand at week 2 after surgery. This is the first rupture out of 300 repairs in the 3 and half years since implementation of this protocol; it happened because the patient did not follow instructions. Otherwise, poor results with severe adhesions or stiffness occurred in 5% of fingers, requiring tenolysis.

VARIATIONS IN PRACTICE AND THEIR RELATIONSHIP TO OUTCOMES

In practice, the surgeons in the 3 units repaired tendons slightly differently from each other, although they all followed the protocol as strictly as they could. After examining intraoperative videos and photographs, slight differences were noted in the surgeons' practice, which is very reasonable and reflects the nature of real-world practice; the techniques used by practicing surgeons, with varying levels of technical proficiency, are often not as "standard" as textbooks would imply.

However, it is intriguing that the surgeons in 3 units obtained outcomes equivalent to the best outcomes reported in the English literature. Reports of surgical details, outcomes, and the analysis of factors affecting outcomes from each of the 3 teams have just begun to appear.[10,11] As they accumulate further cases, we expect other reports in years to come. The details of techniques and outcomes from each team will be included in future reports from the teams. Here we outline a few of their practices, which appear to contradict common teachings; however, despite these technical "flaws," they obtained good outcomes. These findings indicate that those techniques or principles may not be as important as previously believed.

Their Repair Sites are Usually Much Bulkier Than Those of the Lead Author

An often-taught repair principle is to ensure a smooth tendon repair site and to avoid bulkiness. However, according to the results from these units, bulky repairs also lead to good outcomes. The surgeons explained to the lead author that avoiding a bulky repair is difficult in real-world practice. In fact, most surgeons are not very proficient in tendon repair; despite doing their best to avoid a very bulky repair, slightly to moderately bulky repair sites are common and unavoidable in their practice. It is not practical to expect junior surgeons to make as smooth a repair as a very experienced surgeon.

It appears that sufficient tensioning of the repair site through tightening the core suture will always compromise the smoothness of the repair to some degree (**Fig. 4**). Very likely, a slightly or moderately bulky repair is not harmful (or at least not as harmful as previously thought). Because the critical pulleys are vented at the time of surgery, a slightly bulky repair can glide without much difficulty. The repaired tendon tolerates a certain amount of roughness after the pulleys are vented properly. The final outcomes may not be affected by a slightly bulky repair, which is often unavoidable in practice, especially by junior surgeons.

Pulleys Can Be Vented Through a Rather Lengthy Sheath-Pulley Segment, or Sometimes the Entire A2 Pulley if Necessary

Venting a lengthy sheath-pulley or the entire A2 pulley is not recommended. However, some of these surgeons vent the sheath beyond 2 cm, and their patients have not reported bowstringing. Although we do not recommend venting the sheath-pulley longer than 2 cm or the entire A2 pulley, extended venting improves tendon gliding; tendon bowstringing may not be severe enough to cause functional problems. However, this remains an assumption that deserves future investigation. Surgeons should keep in mind that the longer the venting, the greater the risk of tendon bowstringing. There should be a length limit; if not 2.0 cm as suggested previously,[1,5] it might instead be a range (ie, 2.0 to 2.5 cm), but should not exceed 2.5 cm.

Out-of-Splint Motion

The surgeons in these units told the lead author that even though patients actually move more aggressively than instructed, the repairs are strong enough to avoid rupture. These surgeons tend to allow the patients to move rather aggressively. They found that out-of-splint active motion is safe even starting from week 1 or 2. These surgeons have never allowed the patients to move the digits against resistance or move too vigorously when the digits are very swollen and the patients feel marked resistance to motion, which is a key point in instructions to patients.

Not Repairing the Flexor Digitorum Superficialis Tendon Causes No Adverse Outcomes

The surgeons in the 3 units found that not repairing the FDS tendon does not lead to hyperextension of the finger joints. In fact, not repairing the FDS

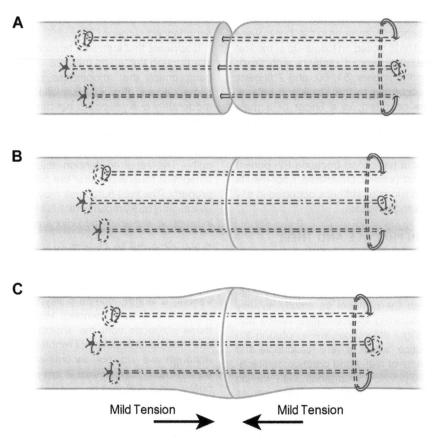

Mild Tension ➡️   ⬅️ Mild Tension

Fig. 4. Bulkiness versus tension across the repair site. (*A*) A loose repair or a repair with gapping should always be avoided. (*B*) Tension-free repair is not an ideal repair. (*C*) Certain bulkiness is always not avoidable in real-world practice. Mild bulkiness at repair site (shown in [*C*]) forming after adding tension to the repair site is not a major problem to tendon gliding with proper pulley-venting. An increase in the repair site diameter by one-fifth to one-fourth is tolerable after completion of the repair, before removal of the temporary fixation needle to the proximal tendon stump. This degree of tension is necessary to ensure no gapping at the repair site during early active digital flexion. *Ensure that tension is not traded for decreasing the bulkiness.* However, remarkable bulkiness at the repair site should always be avoided.

tendon simplifies surgery and makes postoperative finger motion easier. All the surgeons believe that repairing the FDS tendon(s) should not be mandatory and prefer not to repair this tendon when it retracts, the wound is not clean, or if repair is delayed.

The Treatment of Pulleys in the Thumbs Has Not Been Standardized

In the protocol, the methods for pulley treatment in the thumb were not specified, because the literature offers no clear conclusions on which pulleys should be vented. Therefore, surgeons in each unit treat thumb pulleys according to their own preference. All surgeons in these units consider this a topic still awaiting clear guidelines, and anticipate accumulating a larger number of FPL tendon repairs before making any analysis.

Motion Regimen for the Thumb Has Not Been Standardized

The surgeons in each unit instruct patients with an FPL repair to actively flex the thumb with reference to the regimen used in finger tendon repairs. As the thumb differs anatomically from the fingers, the details of exercise instructions to the patients with FPL repairs varied among these surgeons.

OVERALL OUTCOMES AND CONSIDERATIONS

Based on the outcomes in these units, we believe that a multistrand core suture repair, with sufficient release of the sheath and pulley, followed by intraoperative digital extension-flexion, ensures good outcomes. These practices eliminate the risk of repair ruptures when early active motion is practiced appropriately.

We stress that a multistrand repair (for example, 6-strand Tang repair) alone is not sufficient to eliminate the risk of repair rupture. The pulley(s) should be vented to decrease resistance and avoid catching the repair site on the sheath or pulleys. In addition, an intraoperative digital extension-flexion test is especially important for repairs performed by junior surgeons, who should check the quality of the repair via this test. Surgeons must revise their repairs if this test indicates that quality is poor. Therefore, this test is a critical quality check during surgery.

We also suggest that some conventional teachings and suggestions can be revised, because venting of the critical pulleys has become a part of surgery. We believe that the practice of venting the pulleys greatly changes the biomechanics of gliding of a repaired flexor tendon.

Slight Repair Site Bulkiness is Allowed with Tension in Core Suture

The goal of making the repair site as smooth as possible can now be revised: *slight repair site bulkiness is not harmful and can be allowed*. Adding tension to the repair site, a principle not often stressed in the past, should be given sufficient attention and is a technical priority. A strong repair with sufficient tension in the core suture repair, which should be verified through a digital extension-flexion testing, should be key. These 2 measures, adding tension across the repair and performing a digital extension-flexion test, are much more critical than keeping the repair site smooth. Rather, a well-tensioned multistrand repair is beneficial; a multistrand repair without sufficient tension or increased bulk, is harmful. This is not to say that we encourage a bulky repair; a very bulky repair should always be avoided, but a slightly bulky repair causes no hindrance to tendon gliding when the pulleys are properly vented. Surgeons should not trade bulkiness for lack of tension across the repair site. We believe loose sutures without tension are detrimental. Slight bulkiness is neither harmful nor avoidable in the real-world practice of tendon repair.

Wrist Positioning Is No Longer Important

Strong repair methods and pulley-venting decrease the resistance to tendon gliding and increase the ability of the tendon to resist gapping and rupture. We suggest that wrist position is no longer important in postoperative protection. Obviously, one should not place the wrist in marked flexion or marked extension, because both are uncomfortable. Essentially, the patient's wrist can be placed in any position from slight flexion to slight extension; slight flexion to a neutral position appears to be best.

Out-of-Splint Active Motion Is Preferred and Encouraged

Active motion can be performed out of the splint; 1 or 2 weeks after surgery, out-of-splint exercise should be encouraged for efficiency of motion. With the splint's protection, passive extension of the fingers is often insufficient. It becomes hard to achieve "full" extension as required, and splinting adds resistance to active finger flexion, depending on the type and materials of the splint and the amount of dressing on the hand.

PRACTICES IN ASIAN COUNTRIES

In Japan, looped nylon is predominately used to make a tendon repair. The popular method is a Kessler-type 4-strand repair using looped nylon, followed by an additional Tsuge suture repair, making a total 6-strand repair called the Yoshitzu #1 repair.[12,13] Early active flexion is popular. Japanese hand surgeons also vent annular pulleys.[12,13] According to a report, rupture rates of zone 1 and 2 repairs are 6.1% and 5.1%, respectively.[7] In Singapore, a looped nylon suture used to make a 6-strand Lim-Tsai suture is the most frequent method of repairing flexor tendons. In an unpublished audit by Chao and colleagues, the rupture rate was 3% in zone 2 repairs from 2002 to 2007. Both Japanese and Singaporean surgeons have actively performed mechanical studies on repair strength and reported valuable data.[14,15] In Taiwan and Hong Kong, 4-strand repairs are used more often. Surgeons in these regions adopt early active digital flexion and believe the strong repairs in current use can withstand the force of active digital motion.[16] A 2-strand repair has been abandoned for its high rupture rate. Across different regions of the world, surgeons prefer strong core suture repairs.[17-23] Chemical adhesion barriers, barbed sutures, and biological glue are not used.[24-26]

FUTURE PERSPECTIVES

Based on experience from Asian countries, multistrand repairs, especially a 6-strand core suture,[1,7,13,20,27] ensures a strong tendon repair that almost completely prevents repair rupture. Rupture was noted only in rare patients who returned to unrestricted hand use too soon or who had accidents. Venting parts of pulleys is common and considered as important as a strong repair.

Based on findings from 3 surgical centers in this article, it appears that venting the sheath-pulley a bit longer than previously recommended is not harmful and appears to cause no symptomatic tendon bowstringing. Venting can exceed 2 cm if truly needed, although the length limit remains undetermined and apparently varies among fingers and hands of different sizes. Certainly the A2 and A4 pulleys should not both be vented. A report from Japan describes venting the entire A2 pulley in some cases.[13] Canadian surgeons vent the A2 pulley as needed as judged by intraoperative active motion in a wide-awake surgical setting; they do not emphasize keeping even a part of the A2 pulley.[28,29] The best practice for pulley-venting in the thumb is still under question and remains a topic for further research. To evaluate the strength of repair and motion of the tendon, either a passive digital extension-flexion test or active digital extension-flexion test in a wide-awake setting under local anesthesia without a tourniquet[28–32] should be performed routinely.

Early active motion is a popular method in Asia. Out-of-splint motion from the very initial days or the first week of starting exercises is another step forward in pursuing active motion. It is a common impression among many surgeons who use strong repairs that early active motion can be more aggressive than what is currently recommended. Provided no resistance is used and a too-forceful grip is avoided (ie, full active flexion is not attempted), any active motion appears to be safe, with very low rates of rupture. More aggressive pursuit of tendon motion is likely to become a future direction for research. The current strong repairs have given greater freedom to splint-free active motion and more aggressive motion.

Fewer problems are now associated with primary flexor tendon repair than 2 decades ago. Repair rupture does not appear to be a major concern if repair quality has been confirmed through intraoperative digital extension-flexion testing. With early active motion, adhesions are decreased, but tenolysis is still needed in a small percentage of patients; this deserves further investigation. Severe adhesions, although less frequent in clean-cut patients with early active flexion, still develop in the presence of severe trauma or when swelling prohibits adequate passive motion or initiation of active motion. In addition, tendon injuries with loss of a series of major pulleys or tendon defects require secondary pulley and tendon reconstruction.

SUMMARY

The mainstays of Asian practice in primary flexor tendon repair are a strong tendon repair with sufficient venting of the critical pulleys, followed by a combined passive and active exercise program incorporating early active digital flexion. We are moving toward freer active motion, without the protection of a splint during motion exercises; splinting is used between exercise sessions, at a wrist position that patients find comfortable.

REFERENCES

1. Tang JB. Indications, methods, postoperative motion and outcome evaluation of primary flexor tendon repairs in zone 2. J Hand Surg Eur Vol 2007;32:118–29.
2. Elliot D, Giesen T. Primary flexor tendon surgery: the search for a perfect result. Hand Clin 2013;29:191–206.
3. Savage R. The search for the ideal tendon repair in zone 2: strand number, anchor points and suture thickness. J Hand Surg Eur Vol 2014;39:20–9.
4. Tang JB. Outcomes and evaluation of flexor tendon repair. Hand Clin 2013;29:251–9.
5. Tang JB. Release of the A4 pulley to facilitate zone II flexor tendon repair. J Hand Surg Am 2014;39:2300–7.
6. Hoffmann GL, Büchler U, Vögelin E. Clinical results of flexor tendon repair in zone II using a six-strand double-loop technique compared with a two-strand technique. J Hand Surg Eur Vol 2008;33:418–23.
7. Moriya K, Yoshizu T, Maki Y, et al. Clinical outcomes of early active mobilization following flexor tendon repair using the six-strand technique: short- and long-term evaluations. J Hand Surg Eur Vol 2015;40:250–8.
8. Giesen T, Sirotakova M, Copsey AJ, et al. Flexor pollicis longus primary repair: further experience with the Tang technique and controlled active mobilization. J Hand Surg Eur Vol 2009;34:758–61.
9. Tang JB. Tendon surgery. Shanghai: Shanghai Science and Technology Press; 2015.
10. Zhou X, Li XR, Qing J, et al. Outcomes of the 6-strand M-Tang repair for zone 2 primary flexor tendon repair in 54 fingers. J Hand Surg Eur Vol 2017;42:462–8.
11. Pan ZJ, Qing J, Zhou X, et al. Robust thumb flexor tendon repairs with a six-strand M-Tang method, pulley venting, and early active motion. J Hand Surg Eur Vol, in press.
12. Moriya K, Yoshizu T, Tsubokawa N, et al. Outcomes of release of the entire A4 pulley after flexor tendon repairs in zone 2A followed by early active mobilization. J Hand Surg Eur Vol 2016;41:400–5.
13. Moriya K, Yoshizu T, Tsubokawa N, et al. Clinical results of releasing the entire A2 pulley after flexor tendon repair in zone 2C. J Hand Surg Eur Vol 2016;41:822–8.
14. Agrawal AK, Mat Jais IS, Chew EM, et al. Biomechanical investigation of 'figure of 8' flexor tendon repair techniques. J Hand Surg Eur Vol 2016;41:815–21.
15. Kozono N, Okada T, Takeuchi N, et al. Asymmetric six-strand core sutures enhance tendon fatigue strength and the optimal asymmetry. J Hand Surg Eur Vol 2016;41:802–8.
16. Edsfeldt S, Rempel D, Kursa K, et al. In vivo flexor tendon forces generated during different

rehabilitation exercises. J Hand Surg Eur Vol 2015; 40:705–10.

17. Caulfield RH, Maleki-Tabrizi A, Patel H, et al. Comparison of zones 1 to 4 flexor tendon repairs using absorbable and unabsorbable four-strand core sutures. J Hand Surg Eur Vol 2008;33: 412–7.

18. Leppänen OV, Linnanmäki L, Havulinna J, et al. Suture configurations and biomechanical properties of flexor tendon repairs by 16 hand surgeons in Finland. J Hand Surg Eur Vol 2016;41:831–7.

19. Rigo IZ, Røkkum M. Predictors of outcome after primary flexor tendon repair in zone 1, 2 and 3. J Hand Surg Eur Vol 2016;41:793–801.

20. Tang JB. Clinical outcomes associated with flexor tendon repair. Hand Clin 2005;21:199–210.

21. Tang JB, Amadio PC, Boyer MI, et al. Current practice of primary flexor tendon repair: a global view. Hand Clin 2013;29:179–89.

22. Khor WS, Langer MF, Wong R, et al. Improving outcomes in tendon repair: a critical look at the evidence for flexor tendon repair and rehabilitation. Plast Reconstr Surg 2016;138:1045e–58e.

23. Sirotakova M, Elliot D. Early active mobilization of primary repairs of the flexor pollicis longus tendon with two Kessler two-strand core sutures and a strengthened circumferential suture. J Hand Surg Br 2004;29:531–5.

24. O'Brien FP 3rd, Parks BG, Tsai MA, et al. A knotless bidirectional-barbed tendon repair is inferior to conventional 4-strand repairs in cyclic loading. J Hand Surg Eur Vol 2016;41:809–14.

25. Jordan MC, Schmitt V, Dannigkeit S, et al. Surgical adhesive BioGlue™ does not benefit tendon repair strength: an ex vivo study. J Hand Surg Eur Vol 2015;40:700–4.

26. Lees VC, Warwick D, Gillespie P, et al. A multicentre, randomized, double-blind trial of the safety and efficacy of mannose-6-phosphate in patients having zone II flexor tendon repairs. J Hand Surg Eur Vol 2015;40:682–94.

27. Tang JB, Shi D, Gu YQ, et al. Double and multiple looped suture tendon repair. J Hand Surg Br 1994; 19:699–703.

28. Elliot D, Lalonde DH, Tang JB. Commentaries on clinical results of releasing the entire A2 pulley after flexor tendon repair in zone 2C. K. Moriya, T. Yoshizu, N. Tsubokawa, H. Narisawa, K. Hara and Y. Maki. J Hand Surg Eur. 2016, 41: 822–28. J Hand Surg Eur Vol 2016;41:829–30.

29. Lalonde DH. Wide-awake flexor tendon repair. Plast Reconstr Surg 2009;123:623–5.

30. Lalonde D, Higgins A. Wide awake flexor tendon repair in the finger. Plast Reconstr Surg Glob Open 2016;4:e797.

31. Tang JB. Wide-awake primary flexor tendon repair, tenolysis, and tendon transfer. Clin Orthop Surg 2015;7:275–81.

32. Lalonde DH, Martin AL. Wide-awake flexor tendon repair and early tendon mobilization in zones 1 and 2. Hand Clin 2013;29:207–13.

Primary Flexor Tendon Repair with Early Active Motion: Experience in Europe

Thomas Giesen, MD[a],*, Maurizio Calcagni, PD, MD[a],
David Elliot, MA, BM BCh, FRCS[b]

KEYWORDS

- Primary flexor tendon repair • No circumferential suture • Pulley management • FDS resection
- Early active motion

KEY POINTS

- A 6-strand core suture is performed using the M modification of Tang's original technique.
- No circumferential suture is added after a 6-strand core suture.
- The pulleys are divided as much as needed to allow free excursion of the repaired tendon within the tendon sheath, including, when necessary, full division of the A4 or A2 pulley.
- To avoid the repaired structures within the sheath being too bulky, the authors generally repair only half of the flexor digitorum superficialis, resecting the other half. In zone 2C, and in specific cases, the flexor digitorum superficialis is excised completely.
- Rehabilitation is controlled active motion, but with modifications.

INTRODUCTION

Immediate flexor tendon repair of the hand is common practice in European countries. However, routinely achieving a successful outcome from this treatment of flexor tendon lesions in zone 2 has remained an unsolved problem for many decades. Excluding complex cases with associated partial amputation, devascularization or concomitant fractures, immediate repair has traditionally suffered ruptures in approximately 5% of cases and symptomatic adhesions in another 5% of cases, giving unsatisfactory results in 10% of cases.[1]

Various changes of management are being reported worldwide, seeking to reduce these problems and improve results. Both the operative technique and the rehabilitation of

the authors' own protocol have been modified in recent years to try to make the surgery easier and achieve excellent results more regularly.

Alterations of Surgical Technique

These are aims that any suturing technique for flexor tendon repair should include:

- It is simple to perform, particularly by trainees.
- It minimizes tendon manipulation.
- It minimizes the amount of foreign material exposed on the surface of the tendon.
- It provides enough strength for early active mobilization.

Many suturing techniques have been published that attempt to achieve these goals. The authors

The authors have nothing to disclose.
[a] Plastic Surgery and Hand Surgery Division, University Hospital Zurich, Raemistrasse 100, Zurich 8091, Switzerland; [b] St. Andrew's Centre for Plastic Surgery and Burns, Broomfield Hospital, Court Road, Broomfield CM1, UK
* Corresponding author.
E-mail address: Thomas.giesen@usz.ch

hand.theclinics.com

have moved away from the techniques based on the Kessler suture and circumferential suturing, which have dominated practice in Europe for half a century.

The authors currently use the M modification of the Tang technique[2] using a 4-0 loop suture, without circumferential suturing,[3] which the authors believe achieves more of the previously mentioned aims than the more traditional suture techniques.

The authors have also modified management of the tendon sheath, moving away from the belief that the A2 and A4 pulleys are sacrosanct.[4] When necessary, they completely divide one or other. The authors also divide the oblique pulley in the thumb when necessary.

Management of the divided flexor digitorum superficialis (FDS) has also been modified, moving to a policy of partial repair or no repair, depending on the level of FDS division. In selected cases (**Fig. 1**), the authors partially resect the FDS tendon; they resect the FDS completely only when A1 is completely divided, and the lesion is in zone 2C under the A2 pulley. In these cases, the authors do not divide the A2 pulley completely because of the risk of bowstringing. This is based on the evidence that the tendon diameter at a suture site increases by 1.6-fold after repair.[5]

Alterations of Rehabilitation

The authors use a modified controlled active mobilization regime to achieve earlier extension of the wrist, as will be described in the postoperative care section.

CHEMICAL MANIPULATION

The other factor currently being reinvestigated is chemical modification of the tendon and tendon sheath.[6] Until now, this has been by a variety of local chemicals, with limited success, but the future for this avenue of research may lie in manipulation of the growth factors that control tendon healing.

INDICATIONS AND CONTRAINDICATIONS

In the authors' opinion, acute flexor tendon divisions should be repaired within 48 hours. However, late presentation is not uncommon; the authors have all performed delayed primary repair up to 30 days after the injury. Successful delayed primary repair has been reported after much longer delays, even after 1 year.[7] This may require lengthening of the injured tendon proximal to the musculotendinous junction, as described by Le-Viet.[8] Contraindications to delayed repair include infection and significant edema with stiffness in the digit because of a tethering of the extensor

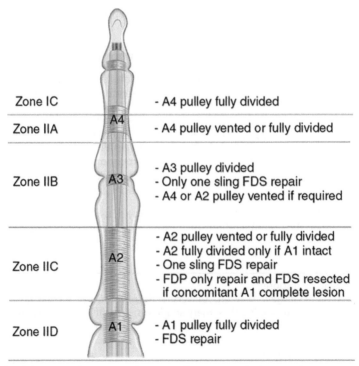

Fig. 1. Zone 1C and subdivisions of zone 2 in fingers and recommended surgical treatments.

tendons. If delayed repair is found to be impossible at surgery because of scarring in the flexor tendon canal or excessive retraction of the proximal stump, the authors would insert a tendon rod as the first stage of a 2-stage tendon graft. The authors personally prefer a 2-stage to a single-stage tendon graft in order to provide an optimal flexor tendon tunnel to the reconstructed tendon, but they are currently considering changing their practice toward a single-stage graft.

SURGICAL PROCEDURES
Preoperative Planning

Local anesthesia in the form of wide-awake surgery[9] is used according to patient wish and compliance and the clinical situation. Otherwise the procedure is performed under brachial block or general anesthesia. If the patient is going to be operated on using wide-awake surgery, the authors still apply a tourniquet to the arm, but without inflating it, in case it is needed during surgery. Although wide-awake surgery has the advantage of allowing one to check that the repair can move through a full range of movement during active flexion and extension, in reality, this can be checked adequately using passive movement of the repair. The main benefit of the newer technique is one of returning anesthesia to the control of the surgeon.

Surgical Approach

The authors routinely use a modified Bruner incision, with the points of the flaps less lateral than the midlateral line in order to avoid necrosis of the tip of the flaps, which would increase scarring. In the thumb, at the metacarpophalangeal (MP) crease, the authors avoid putting the apex of the Bruner incision flap on the ulnar side, as the healing scar may attach to the subcutaneous fibrous tissue of the first web space, causing a web contracture.

Step 1
Contrary to the common practice of classifying the tendon division according to the zone, or subzone, where the tendon sheath has been penetrated, the authors base their decision making on the level of the distal stump of the flexor digitorum profundus (FDP) tendon with the finger fully extended. This identifies the level of the FDP tendon division. In the authors' view, this is a more practical criterion for decision making. Concomitant injuries to the FDS tendon and the nerves and vessels are also noted.

The authors use the Tang subdivisions of zone 2 into subzones 2A to 2D[10] and Elliot's subdivisions

of zone 1 into subzones 1A, 1B, and 1C[11] as a basis for planning subsequent management of the FDP tendon. Although mostly discussing zone 2 injuries, it is sensible to include most zone 1 injuries here, as zone 1B and 1C injuries will also be treated with an intratendinous suture. They will also require venting of the A4 pulley; the 1B repair will catch on the pulley on finger flexion, and the 1C injury lies directly under this pulley and can only be repaired after complete division of the pulley. Decision making about tendon repair and pulley and FDS management is summarized in the flow chart (see **Fig. 1**).

For the thumb, the pulleys are opened sufficiently to perform the repair, but taking care not to completely release both the first pulley and the oblique pulley completely; otherwise there is a risk of appreciable bowstringing.

Step 2
The authors retrieve the proximal stump. When retrieving the proximal stump of the tendon, it is not usually necessary to divide the proximal finger pulleys. If retrieving the proximal stump of the tendon is impossible because of swelling of the tendons, the authors either resect one slip of the FDS and repair only 1 slip or do not repair the FDS at all. If partial FDS repair is carried out, this is done before repairing the FDP tendon. The authors use a single 4-0 loop Tsuge suture; the slip of the FDS that is resected is divided as far proximally as possible to avoid the proximal end catching on the A1 or proximal A2 pulley on finger extension. In the authors' experience, this problem is more likely to arise when attempting delayed primary repair (ie, after 2 days) or when there is more significant trauma to the distal palm or proximal finger than a simple laceration.

The tendon is then manipulated delicately with fine-toothed surgical forceps. Often, only the tendon ends can be held, avoiding gripping the outer surface of the tendon, until a suture has been inserted into the tendon. Thereafter, the tendon is held through the suture. If the surgeon has to grip the surface of a tendon, the authors believe that sharp instruments cause less damage to the tendon than blunt instruments, as the latter do not guarantee a secure grasp of the slippery tendon tissue, leading to multiple attempts at grasping and, therefore, more handling of the tendon.

Step 3
The authors use the M modification of the Tang technique using two 4-0 loop sutures as the core suture of the FDP tendon, as they believe this is an easier technique to master than the Kessler

system.[2] Tang introduced this modification of his original Triple Tsuge technique to reduce the number of loop sutures needed from three to two, for economic reasons. The authors first insert the Tsuge suture into the center of the proximal part of the FDP tendon. Because of the double-barreled nature of the distal part of the FDP tendon, it can be difficult to pass this suture into the center of the distal end, in which case it is inserted into 1 side of the distal tendon end. The authors bury the knots of both sutures in the tendon.

Then, a second loop suture is used to complete the M configuration, placing the 2 strands of the second suture in the dorsal part of the tendon so the load on the repair is dorsal, as this is the part of the tendon mainly stressed in flexion.[12] The authors intentionally let the tendon bulge slightly at the repair site, indicating that more tension than required is being applied, as this ensures good approximation of the tendon stumps. If using a braided looped suture, it is of paramount importance that the tension across the suture is maximized, then maintained, at each step. Otherwise the braided suture may lock before completion of the repair, such that fewer than 6 strands are holding the repair. Monofilament looped sutures are easier to use as they run through the tendon more freely, and this problem does not arise. The authors previously used the 4-0 Fiberloop suture (Arthrex, Naples, Florida) but recently switched to a 4-0 reinforced nylon loop suture. The authors think a 3-0 suture is too bulky.

Traditionally, a circumferential suture was used to tidy the repair and avoid catching. It was later realized that the circumferential suture added strength to the overall repair. The authors believe the tidying process to be unnecessary as the tendon stumps align sufficiently without the circumferential suture. Additional strength is also not needed when a 6-strand core repair is used.[3]

Step 4
Following tendon suture, the repair is moved through a full range of motion, either actively or passively. Any pulley limiting full and free excursion of the repaired tendon is vented or divided as necessary (**Fig. 2**).

Step 5
Repairs of the neurovascular structures are completed, as required, and the skin is closed. A temporary dorsal splint is then made with plaster of Paris and applied with the wrist in neutral and the metacarpophalangeal (MP) joints flexed as much as allowed by the dressings.

POSTOPERATIVE CARE

The principle that immediate mobilization must follow immediate repair was introduced by Kleinert, Verdan, and several others 50 years ago as a sine qua non, without which the fibrin in the edema, described by Watson-Jones in an earlier era as physiological glue, would cause tendon adherence to their surrounds and failure of active tendon and finger movement. Although the degree to which tendon tethering by fibrin occurs may vary between individuals. The authors' protocol is based on the Chelmsford CAM (controlled active motion) regimen of 1994,[13] with several modifications. The

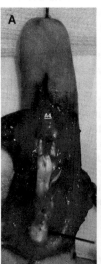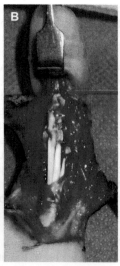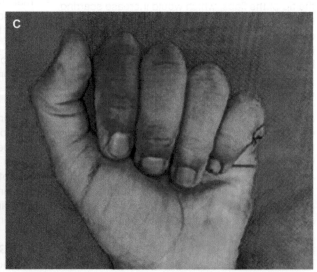

Fig. 2. An FDP tendon repair in the area close to the A4. (*A*) An intact A4 pulley and a disrupted FDP tendon. (*B*) The A4 pulley was entirely divided (*red arrow*) and the FDP tendon was repaired with M-Tang repair method. (*C*) Smooth FDP tendon gliding was confirmed in passive full flexion of the finger during surgery.

protocol highlights briefly the steps taken during the course of hand rehabilitation with the most important message for the patient being that the hand can be mobilized but not used.[14] Other important points not highlighted in the following protocol are early edema control and purposeful patient education.

Days 1 to 5

During these first days

- Dorsal thermoplastic splint should be applied to the whole hand
- Wrist in 20° of extension; metacarpophalangeal joints 40° flexion; interphalangeal joints straight
- During the first 3 weeks the patient is normally seen twice a week by the hand therapists, after this period the frequency is depending on different factors, such as edema, pain, and patient compliance

Week 1

Exercise sessions are carried out hourly, and all exercises are repeated 10 times. The patient starts each exercise session with 10 passive full flexions of the fingers while keeping still wearing the splint. The patient is then allowed to achieve full active finger extension within the splint, followed by active flexion of only 25% of full flexion, using the opposite hand, creating a so-called 3-finger block. Finger flexion is initiated by the FDP.

Week 2

The same regimen is used as for the first week, except that active flexion is taken to 50% of full flexion (2-finger block).

Week 3

The same regimen is used as for the first 2 weeks, except the patient is allowed to perform a full fist without provoking discomfort in form of tension or pain.

Weeks 4 and 5

The patient is allowed to remove the splint and to perform active tenodesis exercises, 10 repetitions, 4 times a day.

Weeks 6 and 7

The patient is seen by the surgeon. The splint is removed during the day, allowing the patient to perform light activities. The splint has to be worn at night and in dangerous situations (eg, in crowds). Progression to full active range of motion of the wrist and fingers continues.

Week 8

Loading exercises are initiated, if it is estimated by the therapist as a 10% difference between passive and active motion of the digits involved; the progression of loading is carefully guided by the hand therapist.[13]

Week 9

The splint is discarded completely. If passive motion is not fully achieved, dynamic splinting is initiated. All but heavy activities are allowed. Driving is allowed. Return to work is allowed for all except heavy manual workers. Return to heavy work is usually allowed from week 12.

Complications

Reduced range of finger movement
Although the injury in these cases is to the palmar surface of the hand, movement of edema onto the dorsum carries fibrin with it, and movement of the digits into flexion is then restricted by fibrin tethering of the extensor tendons. The extensor tendons, moving between interstitial tissue layers and without synovial sheaths, are more susceptible to this problem after any edema-inducing episode in the hand and are responsible for much of the failure of flexor tendon surgery to restore a full range of digital motion. This pathology is far the greatest cause of morbidity after all flexor tendon surgery, wherever and however it is done and whoever does the surgery. The authors try to reduce the edema with antiedema bandage to every finger as soon as the wounds are healed.

Rupture of the repair
In cases of rupture of the repair, the authors reoperate on the patient if he or she returns within 72 hours of rupture. Patients with infection, skin breakdown or swollen, stiff fingers are excluded, as are uncooperative patients. It has been recognized that ruptures of primary repairs of the little finger flexor tendons, albeit with a 2-strand repair, are much more common than ruptures in the other fingers, and second ruptures of rerepairs in this finger are also much more common.[15] It is not known whether this is true for 6-strand core repairs, but technical difficulties, because of the small size of the finger, make use of a 6-strand suture in this finger more difficult, especially after a rupture. If rerepair is found to be impossible, the authors insert a tendon rod as the first stage of a 2-stage tendon grafting procedure.

Flexor tendon adhesion

Fibrin, then scar, adhesion can also occur anywhere along the length of a flexor tendon, with loss of active flexion, but is a particular problem in the fingers themselves, where the flexor tendons are confined within the tendon sheath in a system as finely bored as the pistons in an engine. While this is the third major failure of primary flexor tendon surgery, it gives rise to delayed treatment, and, for the purpose of discussion, falls within the heading of secondary flexor surgery. It is not discussed further in this article.

Hidden rupture of the repair

Although occurring early in the postoperative period after immediate flexor tendon repair, this pathology presents as tendon adhesion. The tendon repair gaps; the tendon is then too long to move through a normal range of motion on activation of the flexor

muscle proximally, and the tendon becomes adherent along its length. The possibility of this pathology being recognized at tenolysis surgery, and the need for converting of the operation from one of tenolysis to one of tendon grafting should be discussed preoperatively with the patient.

The authors are currently achieving no rupture status after primary flexor tendon repair in all cases treated in the manner described. This has been the case for 32 months in 35 FDP tendon repairs in the fingers. However, the authors are still seeing cases requiring tenolysis and do not have 100% good and excellent results.

ROOM FOR IMPROVEMENT
Assessment of Fine Flexor Tendon Function

The authors' means of assessment of flexor tendon repair is far from adequate,[16] and while

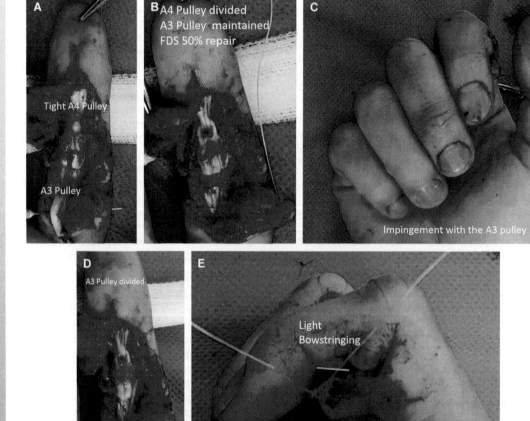

Fig. 3. An example of improving tendon gliding with minor tendon bowstringing at the proximal interphalangeal (PIP) joint level in a zone 2B FDP tendon cut. (*A*) Complete laceration of the FDP tendon at the segment between the A3 and A4 pulleys. (*B*) The A4 pulley was entirely vented. The FDP tendon was repaired with an M-Tang repair; only half of the FDS tendon was repaired, and the A3 pulley was preserved. (*C*) Passive finger flexion cannot fully flex the repaired finger after repair. (*D*) Therefore, the A3 pulley was vented entirely. (*E*) Minor tendon bowstringing noted after venting both the A4 and A3 pulleys.

patient assessments such as the disabilities of the arm, shoulder and hand (DASH) score may be of some additional value, they do not tell any more about the physiology of the flexor tendons and how it is downgraded after tendon repair. This is particularly important at a time when surgery to both the FDS tendon and the tendon sheath is being advocated to accommodate for the bulk of the FDP tendon repair.

The Flexor Digitorum Superficialis Tendon

Although division of half or all of the FDS tendon is being practiced for practical reasons, the precise value to the finger of this tendon remains uncertain. It is possible that this tendon deserves more respect and the bulk of 2 tendon repairs in the fingers be accommodated entirely by modification of the sheath.

The Pulleys

The venting or division of the pulley seems to be the key point to achieve a marked reduction in ruptures rate. The authors have no knowledge of the state of the vented pulleys at the completion of healing. Do they remain vented? Do they heal with lengthening of the pulleys? or do they heal with scar, which contracts, as do all scars, and brings them back to their original size as the tendon repair remodels? The authors are aware from research into the rupture of pulleys among mountain climbers that the pulleys repair in these (closed) cases of rupture if the fingers are mobilized while wearing external circumferential splints on the fingers.[17]

As with modification of the FDS tendon, the assumption that division of the A3 and/or A4 pulleys causes no long-term problems of flexor tendon function[18] is based on relatively crude tests of flexor tendon function (**Fig. 3**). It is possible that finer function of the system is reduced and might be improved by mobilization of the fingers postoperatively in finger ring splints in the hope of pulley repair. The authors are currently investigating whether there is loss of grip strength in digits that have had both the A3 and A4 pulleys completely vented at the same time.

The authors divide the pulleys as much as needed to allow free excursion of the repaired tendon within the tendon sheath, including, when necessary, full division of the A4 or A2 pulley, which is in agreement with the practice and evidence reported in more recent literature that indicate a strong repair should be used,[19–28] as well as critical pulleys vented.[29–38]

SUMMARY

The authors' protocol for primary flexor tendon repair in zones 1 and 2 of the hand is changing to try to make the surgery easier and achieve excellent results more regularly. This article discusses some of the changes made recently. The authors now perform an immediate repair within 48 hours whenever possible but have operated on suitable cases up to 1 month after injury. The authors perform a 6-strand core suture using the M modification of Tang's original technique, with no circumferential suture. They divide the pulleys as much as needed to allow free excursion of the repaired tendon within the tendon sheath, including, when necessary, full division of the A4 or A2 pulley. To avoid the repaired structures within the sheath being too bulky, the authors also, mostly, repair only half of the FDS, resecting the other half. In zone 2C, and in specific cases, the authors excise the FDS completely. Rehabilitation remains based on controlled active motion,[15,39] but with modifications.

ACKNOWLEDGMENTS

The authors would like to thank Vera Beckmann-Fries and the Hand Therapy Department of the University Hospital Zurich for their contribution.

REFERENCES

1. Elliot D, Giesen T. Primary flexor tendon surgery: the search for a perfect result. Hand Clin 2013;29: 191–206.
2. Wang B, Xie RG, Tang JB. Biomechanical analysis of a modification of Tang method of tendon repair. J Hand Surg Br 2003;28:347–50.
3. Giesen T, Sirotakova M, Copsey AJ, et al. Flexor pollicis longus primary repair: further experience with the tang technique and controlled active mobilization. J Hand Surg Eur Vol 2009;34:758–61.
4. Rigo IZ, Røkkum M. Predictors of outcome after primary flexor tendon repair in zone 1, 2 and 3. J Hand Surg Eur Vol 2016;41:793–801.
5. Puippe GD, Lindenblatt N, Gnannt R, et al. Prospective morphologic and dynamic assessment of deep flexor tendon healing in zone II by high-frequency ultrasound: preliminary experience. Am J Roentgenol 2011;197:W1110–7.
6. Tang JB, Wu YF, Cao Y, et al. Gene therapy for tendon healing. In: Tang JB, Amadio PC, Guimberteau JC, et al, editors. Tendon surgery of the hand. Philadelphia: Elsevier Saunders; 2012. p. 59–70.
7. McFarlane RM, Lamon R, Jarvis G. Flexor tendon injuries within the finger. A study of the results of tendon suture and tendon graft. J Trauma 1968;8: 987–1003.
8. Le Viet D. Flexor tendon lengthening by tenotomy at the musculotendinous junction. Ann Plast Surg 1986;17:239–46.

9. Lalonde DH, Martin AL. Wide-awake flexor tendon repair and early tendon mobilization in zones 1 and 2. Hand Clin 2013;29:207–13.

10. Tang JB. Outcomes and evaluation of flexor tendon repair. Hand Clin 2013;29:251–9.

11. Moiemen NS, Elliot D. Primary flexor tendon repair in zone 1. J Hand Surg Br 2000;25:78–84.

12. Tang JB, Pan CZ, Xie RG, et al. A biomechanical study of Tang's multiple locking techniques for flexor tendon repair. Chir Main 1999;18:254–60.

13. Elliot D, Moiemen NS, Flemming AF, et al. The rupture rate of acute flexor tendon repairs mobilized by the controlled active motion regimen. J Hand Surg Br 1994;19:607–12.

14. Higgins A, Lalonde DH. Flexor tendon repair postoperative rehabilitation: the Saint John Protocol. Plast Reconstr Surg Glob Open 2016;4:e1134.

15. Groth GN. Pyramid of progressive force exercises to the injured flexor tendon. J Hand Ther 2004;17:31–42.

16. Elliot D, Harris SB. The assessment of flexor tendon function after primary tendon repair. Hand Clin 2003;19:495–503.

17. Schreiber T, Allenspach P, Seifert B, et al. Connective tissue adaptations in the fingers of performance sport climbers. Eur J Sport Sci 2015;15:696–702.

18. Franko OI, Lee NM, Finneran JJ, et al. Quantification of partial or complete A4 pulley release with FDP repair in cadaveric tendons. J Hand Surg Am 2011;36:439–45.

19. Leppänen OV, Linnanmäki L, Havulinna J, et al. Suture configurations and biomechanical properties of flexor tendon repairs by 16 hand surgeons in Finland. J Hand Surg Eur Vol 2016;41:831–7.

20. Hoffmann GL, Büchler U, Vögelin E. Clinical results of flexor tendon repair in zone II using a six-strand double-loop technique compared with a two-strand technique. J Hand Surg Eur Vol 2008;33:418–23.

21. Moriya K, Yoshizu T, Maki Y, et al. Clinical outcomes of early active mobilization following flexor tendon repair using the six-strand technique: short- and long-term evaluations. J Hand Surg Eur Vol 2015;40:250–8.

22. Edsfeldt S, Rempel D, Kursa K, et al. In vivo flexor tendon forces generated during different rehabilitation exercises. J Hand Surg Eur Vol 2015;40:705–10.

23. Tang JB. Clinical outcomes associated with flexor tendon repair. Hand Clin 2005;21:199–210.

24. Savage R, Tang JB. History and nomenclature of multistrand repairs in digital flexor tendons. J Hand Surg Am 2016;41:291–3.

25. Savage R. The search for the ideal tendon repair in zone 2: strand number, anchor points and suture thickness. J Hand Surg Eur Vol 2014;39:20–9.

26. Kozono N, Okada T, Takeuchi N, et al. Asymmetric six-strand core sutures enhance tendon fatigue strength and the optimal asymmetry. J Hand Surg Eur Vol 2016;41:802–8.

27. Agrawal AK, Mat Jais IS, Chew EM, et al. Biomechanical investigation of 'figure of 8' flexor tendon repair techniques. J Hand Surg Eur Vol 2016;41:815–21.

28. O'Brien FP 3rd, Parks BG, Tsai MA, et al. A knotless bidirectional–barbed tendon repair is inferior to conventional 4-strand repairs in cyclic loading. J Hand Surg Eur Vol 2016;41:809–14.

29. Elliot D, Lalonde DH, Tang JB. Commentaries on clinical results of releasing the entire A2 pulley after flexor tendon repair in zone 2C. K. Moriya, T. Yoshizu, N. Tsubokawa, H. Narisawa, K. Hara and Y. Maki. J Hand Surg Eur 2016, 41: 822–28. J Hand Surg Eur Vol 2016;41:829–30.

30. Moriya K, Yoshizu T, Tsubokawa N, et al. Outcomes of release of the entire A4 pulley after flexor tendon repairs in zone 2A followed by early active mobilization. J Hand Surg Eur Vol 2016;41:400–5.

31. Moriya K, Yoshizu T, Tsubokawa N, et al. Clinical results of releasing the entire A2 pulley after flexor tendon repair in zone 2C. J Hand Surg Eur Vol 2016;41:822–8.

32. Zhou X, Li QR, Qing J, et al. Outcomes of the 6-strand M-Tang repair for zone 2 primary flexor tendon repair in 54 fingers. J Hand Surg Eur Vol 2017;42:462–8.

33. Tang JB. Indications, methods, postoperative motion and outcome evaluation of primary flexor tendon repairs in Zone 2. J Hand Surg Eur Vol 2007;32:118–29.

34. Tang JB. Release of the A4 pulley to facilitate zone II flexor tendon repair. J Hand Surg Am 2014;39:2300–7.

35. Tang JB, Chang J, Elliot D, et al. IFSSH Flexor Tendon Committee report 2014: from the IFSSH Flexor Tendon Committee. J Hand Surg Eur Vol 2014;39:107–15.

36. Tang JB, Amadio PC, Boyer MI, et al. Current practice of primary flexor tendon repair: a global view. Hand Clin 2013;29:179–89.

37. Wong JK, Peck F. Improving results of flexor tendon repair and rehabilitation. Plast Reconstr Surg 2014;134:913e–25e.

38. Khor WS, Langer MF, Wong R, et al. Improving outcomes in tendon repair: a critical look at the evidence for flexor tendon repair and rehabilitation. Plast Reconstr Surg 2016;138:1045e–58e.

39. Elliot D. Primary flexor tendon repair–operative repair, pulley management and rehabilitation. J Hand Surg Br 2002;27:507–13.

The Nonoperative Management of Hand Fractures in United Kingdom

Grey Giddins, FRCS (Orth), EDHS

KEYWORDS

- Hand fractures • Metacarpal fracture • Spiral fracture • Transverse fracture • Avulsion fracture
- Mallet finger

KEY POINTS

- Spiral or long oblique metacarpal fractures, metacarpal neck fractures, and bony collateral ligament injuries of the finger and thumb MP joints do so well with nonoperative treatment that there is rarely a role for surgery.
- Bennett fractures may be successfully treated nonoperatively; surgery should not be the only option.
- Assessment of gliding or pivoting in intra-articular fractures of the bases of the middle (fracture subluxations and pilon fractures) and distal (bony mallet injuries) phalanges helps to identify those fractures likely to do well enough not to need surgery.

INTRODUCTION

One hundred years ago hand fractures were virtually always treated nonoperatively (conservatively). Over the last 50 years surgical treatment of some hand fractures has become popular. This is typically with Kirschner(K) wires or internal fixation, the latter led by the AO group.[1] Although K wiring or open reduction and internal fixation (ORIF) and their many variants can be used to treat any hand fracture, this does not mean they should. It is easy for clinicians and patients to be misled by the purported advantages of surgery. A case series reporting good results may be presented or published and surgeons may believe that that technique should be followed. Yet most hand fractures do well with nonoperative treatment.[2] Therefore even relatively unsuccessful surgical treatment, such as malunion following K wiring or ORIF, may still give a good outcome.

In the United Kingdom medical care has largely been provided within the National Health Service (NHS) especially for treatment of injuries and emergencies. The doctors are paid a salary independent of treatment removing any incentive to operative to improve remuneration. In addition the NHS has been chronically underfunded (ie, underresourced), encouraging staff to adopt less resource-intensive treatment, such as conservative rather than operative treatment. Therefore there has been a much greater emphasis on nonoperative treatment of hand fractures in the United Kingdom than in some other countries. This may sometimes cause undertreatment and acceptance of poorer results. All treatment decisions should be justifiable based on current best evidence.

This article identifies the fractures that are still best treated nonoperatively. A secondary aim is to establish where there may be subgroups of those fractures requiring surgery that have not been defined.

LITERATURE REVIEW

I performed multiple electronic and subsequent hand searches of published literature to identify fractures that do so well with nonoperative treatment that it is currently too difficult for surgery to

The author has nothing to disclose.
The Hand to Elbow Clinic, 29a James Street West, Bath BA1 2BT, UK
E-mail address: greygiddins@thehandclinic.co.uk

Hand Clin 33 (2017) 473–487
http://dx.doi.org/10.1016/j.hcl.2017.04.006
0749-0712/17/Crown Copyright © 2017 Published by Elsevier Inc. All rights reserved.

provide significant further benefit. The inclusion criteria were as follows: all adult (≥16 years of age) fractures of the hand, excluding carpal injuries; papers that had a minimum of five cases; and I planned only to include papers with a minimum follow-up of 2 years. This proved impractical because so few had such adequate follow-up and so all papers with a minimum follow-up of 6 weeks were included. Even then reports often had patients less than 16 years old, which could not be separated out. The exclusion criteria were fractures where surgery is plainly needed and proven to have been beneficial: many open fractures, replantations, many crush injuries, displaced intra-articular fractures (excluding bony mallet injuries and ligament avulsion fractures), and pediatric fractures.

TREATMENT OF FRACTURES IN THE HAND
Spiral or Long Oblique Metacarpal Fractures

The spiral or long oblique fractures of the metacarpals are common (**Fig. 1**). They can be treated surgically; various techniques have been described and good results have been reported.[3–5] Similar good results have been reported with nonoperative treatment.[6] Recently Khan and Giddins[7] have shown that all spiral metacarpal fractures, even in the presence of initial malrotation, can be treated nonoperatively with excellent or very good outcomes and minimal morbidity (**Table 1**). All patients were treated with early mobilization, without a splint or plaster. They were encouraged to "make a fist" at the first hand clinic visit to

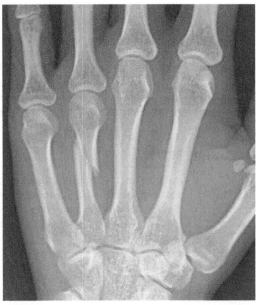

Fig. 1. An oblique fracture of the metacarpal bone.

correct any malrotation and ensure early mobilization. Twenty-five of 30 patients were reviewed at a minimum of 6 months. They had full, painless movement and grip strength of at least 90% of the other hand. The only adverse problems were minimal malrotation in one patient and mild discomfort in another.

Previous authors have been concerned by the risk of hand dysfunction caused by shortening of the metacarpals following nonoperative treatment[8–10]; a recent study has suggested that shortening up to 5 mm is not biomechanically significant.[11] This fits with the results of the study of Khan and Giddins.[7] They confirmed that the metacarpals derotate through tightening of the intermetacarpal ligaments, which also limit shortening to 2 to 5 mm. Their results confirm that this degree of shortening is not typically clinically relevant.

Malrotation following spiral metacarpal fractures almost always corrects with finger flexion. If it does not, then encouragement or (rarely) manipulation under local anesthetic is appropriate because a key aim of treatment is avoidance of rotational malunion. Nonoperative treatment gives such good results that recommending surgery seems unjustifiable in almost all patients.

Finger Transverse Metacarpal Fractures: Shaft and Neck

In the past virtually all patients with transverse metacarpal shaft and particularly neck (boxer's) fractures were encouraged to mobilize freely; patients healed with some deformity but almost always good function. In the United Kingdom, Barton[2] in particular showed the benefits of plaster or splint support to reduce and successfully maintain an improved angulation for transverse metacarpal shaft fractures. More recently the results of surgical treatments have been reported with good results.

A crucial question is: what degree of metacarpal malunion is acceptable? The answer is not clear. For metacarpal neck (boxer's) fractures it has been suggested by various authors as 50° to 60° flexion,[12] 30°,[13,14] and 20°.[15,16] It is noticeable that the amount of acceptable angulation has increased over time. For little finger metacarpal shaft fractures 30°[12,17] has been suggested as acceptable. These recommendations are only expert opinion.

The outcome of nonoperative treatment has been reported widely and apart from a mild cosmetic abnormality, there is typically an excellent functional outcome.[18] A Cochrane review has noted that there is no good evidence that more marked malunion reduces hand function

Table 1
The outcomes of finger spiral or long oblique metacarpal fractures in literature

Authors and Year	Treatments	Numbers of Patients (Fingers)	Mean Follow-up (Range), mo	Mean Age (Range), y	Ranges of Motion	Grip Strength	Complications
Al-Qattan,[4] 2008	Cerclage wiring and interosseous loop wiring	24 (25)	2.5 (1.5–7)	32 (20–42)	Full in 23		CRPS in 1
Al-Qattan,[6] 2008	Splint and mobilization	42 (54)	Min 1.5 Max 12	29 (20–48)		94% in those seen at 1 y	
Al-Qattan & Al-Lazzam,[5] 2007	Cerclage wire	19	2 (1.5–3)	35 (18–45)	Full		None
Khan & Giddins,[7] 2015	Early mobilization	25 (28)	Min 6 (range 6–14)	27 (17–60)	Full	>90% in all	Mild malrotation in one Mild discomfort in a boxer

Abbreviation: CRPS, complex regional pain syndrome.

or gives an unacceptable deformity.[18] More marked deformities may give functional problems; if proven this would suggest a role for surgery where the deformity could not be reduced adequately using nonoperative techniques.

Many surgical techniques have been described including intramedullary nailing,[19] intramedullary screw fixation,[20–22] K-wire (bouquet) fixation,[23–25] intraosseous loop wire fixation,[3] and external fixation.[26] The results of these techniques are not reliably better than nonoperative treatment and they introduce complications not seen with nonoperative treatment. Nonoperative treatment has complications. Apart from malunion these are rare. They are primarily related to immobilization in a plaster or splint.

Comparative studies, particularly randomized controlled studies (RCTs), offer the best way to assess different treatments. In hand surgery excellent RCTs are rare but there are some useful comparative studies. Westbrook and colleagues[27] compared nonsurgical and surgical treatment of metacarpal neck and shaft fractures in a retrospective study. They reported on metacarpal neck and shaft fractures: 105 metacarpal neck fractures were treated nonoperatively compared with 18 treated operatively (intramedullary K wiring in 13 and plating in five cases); and 113 metacarpal shaft fractures were treated nonoperatively compared with 26 treated operatively (K wiring in four and plating in 22 cases). At a minimum

follow-up of 2 years there were no differences in DASH (Disability of Arm Shoulder and Hand) score, grip strengths, or aesthetics between the nonoperative and operative groups. But there was a significantly higher complication rate in the patients treated operatively compared with those treated nonoperatively. The follow-up rates were low (17% for nonoperative treatment and 54% for operative treatment) as is typical in these patient groups. A randomized study of the treatment of metacarpal neck fractures by Strub and colleagues[28] has suggested that surgery may give slightly better outcomes than nonoperative treatment, primarily giving a better cosmetic result because of less malunion. In this study there were two groups each of 20 patients who were pseudorandomized. The patients receiving surgery were treated with intramedullary (bouquet) wiring. They required a minimum of two operations each; one to insert and one to remove the wires. The only complications were in the operative group; they also had more dissatisfied and more very satisfied patients. This study did not take into account the inconvenience and costs to the patient or the health care system, so the cost of this possible small benefit is not known. In addition it is not clear how many patients need to be improved from "satisfied" to "very satisfied" to compensate for one "dissatisfied" patient.

Overall there may be a small cosmetic benefit from surgery for transverse metacarpal shaft and neck fractures but the costs and the risks are probably not worth the small potential benefit to most patients and in particular most health care systems, especially the NHS.

Finger Proximal Phalanx Collateral Ligament Avulsion Fractures

Bekler and colleagues[29] noted that avulsion fractures of the bases of the phalanges are challenging injuries to treat (**Fig. 2**); they also stated that "avulsion fractures (of the bases of the phalanges) are intra-articular according to their configuration and need anatomic reduction." There was no evidence to support this opinion. Despite this confident assertion proximal phalanx avulsion fractures are a group of injuries that attract a full range of proven treatment advice.

Many authors have recommended that all base of finger avulsion fractures be treated surgically because of the high rate of symptomatic nonunion or delayed union.[30–35] Shewring and Thomas[35] reported that of eight of their patients treated nonoperatively all had delayed union; seven were treated with open reduction, screw fixation, and bone grafting. They reported good results at 3 months following surgery. However, as also reported in the United Kingdom, finger proximal phalanx avulsion fractures of up to 25% of the articular surface on the posteroanterior radiograph achieve reliable results with early protected mobilization.[36] Overall,

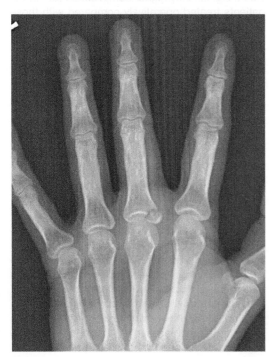

Fig. 2. An avulsion fracture at the base of the proximal phalanx.

for avulsion fractures protected mobilization gives results that cannot easily be improved by surgery (**Table 2**). The available data are, however, limited either because these are small series or have limited follow-up. The dichotomy with the experience of Shewring and Thomas[35] who reported symptomatic delayed union in eight consecutive patients and the excellent results of Sawant and colleagues[36] may be that many of these injuries do not unite with bone (as for thumb metacarpophalangeal [MP] joint ulnar collateral ligament [UCL] avulsions)[37] but heal with sufficient stability that surgery is not required.

Thumb Metacarpophalangeal Joint Avulsion Fractures

Ulnar collateral ligament injuries

The outcome of thumb MP joint avulsion fractures (**Fig. 3**) treated nonoperatively is also disputed. It is clearly understood that the presence of a Stener lesion, whether or not there is a bony avulsion, almost always gives a poor long-term outcome with nonoperative treatment[38]; therefore surgery should be performed for these patients.

For less displaced injuries without a Stener lesion some authors have reported poor outcomes of avulsion fractures treated nonoperatively: Dinowitz and colleagues[39] reported on nine cases with minimally displaced fractures (up to 2 mm) treated in plaster within 6 days. They reported that all had persistent pain, which largely resolved with surgical stabilization. Kuz and colleagues[40] reported on 30 patients who were satisfied by their treatment and none had had to change their jobs. Of the 20 patients assessed in person there was no statistically significant reduction in pinch or grip strength but two patients had some instability on stress testing. The nonunion rate was 5 of 20. Sorene and Goodwin[37] reported on 28 patients with thumb UCL avulsion fractures that were stable at original assessment. The patients were treated with immobilization in plaster for 6 weeks and followed up for a mean of 2.5 (range 1–4) years. Twenty-six of the 28 patients were pain-free and all patients had the same pinch and grip strength as their contralateral uninjured side, yet 60% had radiologic evidence of persistent nonunion of the fracture fragment. Comparable good results have been reported by other authors.[30,41] Stable thumb UCL bony avulsion injuries can be immobilized in plaster with the expectation of a good clinical outcome even though radiologic union may not be achieved (**Table 3**).

The treatment of unstable thumb MP joint UCL avulsion injuries is less clear; at present surgery is probably the default position, but because the

Table 2
The outcome of finger proximal phalanx avulsion fractures

Authors and Year	Treatment	Numbers of Patients (Fingers)	Mean Follow-up (Range), mo	Mean Age (Range), y	Function DASH Scores	Ranges of Motion	Grip Strength
Sawant et al,[36] 2007	Early mobilization	7 (7)	57 (8–94)	39 (16–68)	1.3 (0–4.2)	Full	>90%
Mikami et al,[33] 2011	K wiring	4 (5)	43 (30–72)	21 (11–57)	3.0 (0.8–10.8)	85°	—
Shewring & Thomas,[35] 2003	Open reduction and internal fixation	33	3	26 (15–44)	—	Full	—

data often are inadequate. There are many different types of thumb UCL avulsion injury from small bony avulsions, which seem primarily to be a soft tissue problem through to large rotated bone avulsion fragments. It is highly likely this is an injury with subtypes requiring different treatment; some may do appreciably better treated surgically, whereas most may not. This remains unproven, but it would in part explain the dichotomy between the advocates of nonoperative and operative treatment.

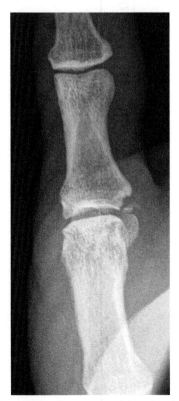

Fig. 3. An avulsion fracture involving the thumb MP joint.

An adequately powered (probably quite large study to identify the subtypes) multicenter RCT is needed. Although nonoperative management should remain the treatment of choice for thumb MP joint UCL bony avulsion fractures, surgeons need to be aware that there is a range of injuries that may be treated differently.

Radial collateral ligament injuries

There are fewer reports of the treatment of radial collateral ligament (RCL) injuries. Because there is no adductor hood to give a Stener-type lesion nonoperative treatment should give good results; that is, immobilization in plaster or a splint for 4 to 6 weeks. Despite this, surgical treatment of these injuries has been debated for a long time.[42–45] There are also rare reports of radial-sided Stener lesions.[46,47]

Kottstorfer and colleagues[48] showed that mildly displaced RCL avulsion fractures treated nonoperatively usually achieve a good outcome. The role of surgery for more widely displaced or unstable injuries is unclear. Kottstorfer and colleagues[48] noted that many surgeons believe that surgery is required for unstable injuries as "considerable displacement of torn ends can prevent the RCL from healing." Good results have been reported with surgical stabilization for more unstable injuries, but the original premise that the ligament will not heal with marked displacement or instability is unproven. In addition it is well known that in the hand considerable ligament disruption can usually be repaired by the body's own mechanisms avoiding instability. One reason for the different clinical approaches may be the long time to recover fully from thumb MP joint radial and UCL avulsion injuries. This may skew the clinical impression of treatment outcome in shorter-term reviews.

RCL injuries vary greatly; the optimal treatment for each subgroup is not yet established but again

Table 3
Thumb MP Joint ulnar collateral ligament bony avulsions

Authors and Year	Treatment	Number of Patients (Thumbs)	Mean Follow-up (Range), mo	Mean Age (Range), y	Ranges of MP Joint Movement, %	Grip Strength, %	Notes
Kozin & Bishop,[41] 1994	Tension band wiring	9	26	20 (15–41)	77	96	
Kuz et al,[40] 1999	Plaster cast or splint for 4 wk	30	3.1 (1–5.2)	30	The same	—	No pain in 19/30 Unstable in 2/20 Nonunion 5/20
Landsman et al,[85] 1995	Thumb spica splint for 8–12 wk	12	38 (12–60)	30 (17–48)	84 (60–100)	92 (80–100)	All healed but data on range of motion and strength includes tendinous injuries, which overall did worse than the avulsion injuries
Sorene & Goodwin,[37] 2003	Plaster cast	28	30 (12–48)	34 (17–62)	—	97	No pain in 26 Nonunion 17

nonoperative treatment should be presumed to be the management of choice for most of these injuries.

Bony Mallet Injuries

There have been a multitude of papers reporting on a myriad of techniques for reducing and holding the dorsal avulsion fracture fragment in bony mallet injuries.[49–62] This is an operation with an acknowledged high risk of complications.[30,63,64] Authors of more recent techniques report a lower risk of complications particularly the risks of skin breakdown.[49–62] In general good results are reported for various surgical treatments of bony mallet injuries with a dorsal fracture fragment of one-third or more (**Table 4**). The recommendation to treat fractures of one-third or more has come from several authors especially Stark and colleagues.[67] They and other authors have been concerned about achieving "anatomic reduction" of the fracture and preventing subluxation of the main distal phalanx fracture fragment.[50–62] When subluxation needs to be treated is unproven, although some cases do progress to symptomatic dislocation.

Webhe and Schneider[64] reported that 15 patients treated nonoperatively did as well as the six treated operatively. They concluded that operative treatment gave no better results than nonoperative treatment. Similarly a series with a 5-year follow-up has shown that tendinous and bony mallet injuries treated nonoperatively achieve good objective and good subjective outcomes. Among the bony mallet injuries were some with fracture fragments greater than one-third but they are not reported separately. They also reported some evidence of degeneration at the distal inter-phaangeal (DIP) joint in 10 of 11 patients with large fracture fragments within 5 years. Other authors have reported on degeneration. Webhe and Schneider[64] noted no difference between operative and nonoperative treatment in rates of radiographic osteoarthritis (OA). Other authors have reported rates up to 50%, yet some of only 0% (see **Table 4**). Almost certainly their criteria (which are reported rarely) differ, making comparison difficult.

The risk of radiographic OA is a potential concern. However, long-term symptomatic degenerative arthritis in the DIP joints is not widely reported in patients who have had bony mallet injuries. Hand surgeons rarely see patients requiring treatment of symptomatic DIP joint arthritis who had bony mallet injuries decades earlier. Most patients with bony mallet injuries do not require surgical treatment.

A Cochrane review reported that there was a paucity of good studies and there was no evidence that surgery was better than nonoperative (typically splint) treatment of all types of mallet injury.[68] They did, however, acknowledge that there may be a subgroup of these injuries that would benefit from surgery.

The main area of concern is when there is a large fracture fragment greater than one-third of the articular surface on the lateral radiograph, which may lead to volar subluxation of the main distal fracture fragment of the distal phalanx. Several recent papers have clarified further the risk of subluxation. Kim and Kim[68] showed that more than 50% of patients with a fracture fragment involving greater than one-third of the base on the lateral radiograph did not progress to subluxation. They noted a cutoff of a fracture fragment size of 48% of the base, above which subluxation was more likely. This is also similar to the findings in the study of Giddins[69] who noted that stable injuries had a mean fracture fragment size of 49%. Kim and Kim[68] also related subluxation to delay in application of a splint, particularly to a delay of longer than 12 days. Moradi and colleagues[70] reviewed 392 bony mallet injuries. They showed that subluxation did not occur with a fracture fragment smaller than 39% on the lateral radiograph. The risk of subluxation increased with increasing size of the fragment, increased displacement of the fragment, and time from injury to treatment. Nonetheless most (68%) did not sublux even with a fracture fragment greater than 39%. Giddins[69] has shown that the risk of subluxation is assessed by a lateral hyperextension radiograph performed within 1 to 2 weeks of injury.

If there is gliding of the joint (**Fig. 4**), that is, it remains congruent as it goes into extension, then this is a stable joint. The presumption is that there has not been so much collateral ligament injury that subluxation occurs. If there is pivoting (**Fig. 5**) then subluxation usually occurs, although this may only be mild. A third subgroup occurs called tilting (**Fig. 6**). This seems to be a variant on gliding and is not typically associated with subluxation. Exactly what level of subluxation requires treatment is unclear. Together these papers clearly establish that using the criteria of a fracture fragment greater than one-third of the base of the distal phalanx is unreliable in predicting subluxation and so recommending surgery. Rather, a combination of the fracture fragment size greater than 39%, displacement, and particularly the response to hyperextension testing should indicate the small number of patients who require surgery to prevent appreciable, long-term symptomatic subluxation. Most should do well with

Table 4
The outcome of treatment of bony mallet injuries with fracture fragments greater than or equal to one-third and a minimum follow-up of 12 months

Authors and Year	Treatment	Numbers of Patients (Fingers)	Mean FU (Range), mo	Mean Age (Range), y	DIP Joint Ranges of Motion (Degrees)	% of Bone Involved on the Lateral Radiograph	Crawford (or Other) Score	Radiologic Evidence of Osteoarthritis
Damron & Engber,[53] 1994	Pull-through suture and K wire	18	97 (24–147)	23 (17–32)	1–69 (15 patients)	51 (38–67)	10 pain-free, 13 no functional limitation	7/15
Darder-Prats et al,[54] 1998	K wire	22	25 (18–48)	23 (14–34)	NR	>33	18 E, 3 G, 1 F	0
Fritz et al,[55] 2005	K wire	24	Mean unclear (min 12 mo)	31 (15–53)	1–72	>33	19 no pain W and N criteria	
Okafor et al,[65,66] 1997	Splint for 7 (6–12) wk	11	66 (but also includes tendinous)	—	9–51	—	—	10/11
Hofmeister et al,[86] 2003	Closed K wiring	23 (24)	>1 y	24	4–77	40	22 E/G, 2 F	
Takami et al,[87] 2000	Open reduction and K wiring	33	29	32 (19–63)	4–67	>33	—	
Tetik & Gudemez,[88] 2002	Closed K wiring	18	27	29 (22–47)	2–81	40	—	

Abbreviations: E, excellent; F, fair; G, good.

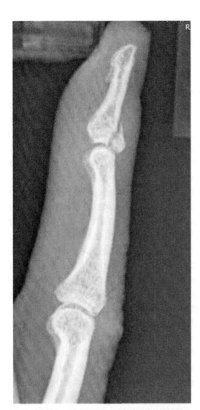

Fig. 4. Bony mallet gliding with hyperextension stress testing.

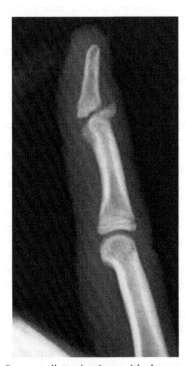

Fig. 5. Bony mallet pivoting with hyperextension stress testing.

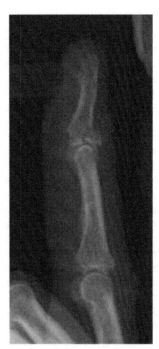

Fig. 6. Bony mallet tilting with hyperextension stress testing.

splintage. The recent work on this injury is helping define the subgroups where surgery is indicated and helping exclude more patients from needing operations.

Bennett Fracture Subluxation

The treatment of Bennett fracture subluxations has move from a clear preference for nonoperative treatment 30 or more years ago to a consistent preference for surgical stabilization (percutaneous or open and with many different techniques) such that statements are published that conservative treatment is less good than operative treatment. Whether this is proven by the published literature in not clear.

A recent systematic review looked at the evidence in the treatment of Bennett fractures.[71] Thirty-eight different retrospective studies were reviewed; they were published from 1958 to 2015. There were 11 different types of treatment from immobilization for only 1 week to ORIF. The reporting of data was not consistent preventing a meta-analysis. Nonetheless it was possible to compare the outcomes for hundreds of patients. Pain was reported in 31 studies, return to work in 28 studies, and radiologic evidence of OA in 31 studies. Long-term assessment of pain could be compared for 645 patients: 75 of 224 (33%) patients treated nonsurgically had pain at final review (mean time, 12; range, 6–26 years), compared with 73 of 421 (17%) treated surgically (mean time, 5; range, 2–11 years) (P<.0001). Data on return to work could be compared for 474 patients. A total of 120 of 122 (98%) patients treated nonsurgically returned to their previous employment at a mean of 11 (range, 2–26) years, compared with 351 of 352 (99%) of those treated surgically at a mean of 6 (range, 1–12) years. Radiologic evidence of OA was reported in 839 patients: 99 of 299 (33%) patients treated nonsurgically had OA at a mean of 8 (range, 2–26) years, compared with 182 of 540 (33%) patients treated surgically at a mean of 4 (range, 1–12) years. Data on complications of treatment were available for 956 patients; only 2 of 287 (<1%) of patients treated nonsurgically had complications compared with 88 of 669 (13%) treated surgically; 56 patients of the latter group required a second operation for removal of prominent tension band wires (P = .0001).

The quality of the data is not high. Nonetheless it seems that patients are more likely to suffer long-term pain following nonsurgical treatment and much more likely to suffer complications with surgical treatment. Otherwise the data for return to work and long-term OA are comparable.

The longest review (mean, 26 years) is from Livesley.[72] It is frequently cited as evidence for treating these injuries operatively rather than non-operatively.[73] Yet in Livesley's cohort of 17 patients, no comment is made on the quality of the reduction at the beginning of treatment and three different methods of treatment were used: no immobilization in two cases, traction in four, and manipulation and plaster in 11. At the final review 11 of the 17 had no or mild pain and 16 of the 17 had returned to their previous employment. Furthermore, although this paper has the longest follow-up, when degenerative changes may be expected to lead to symptoms, their results are not significantly different in terms of pain and function to similar conservative studies and perhaps more importantly to several of the operative studies.[74–77]

Overall there is currently no high-quality evidence as to the optimal treatment method for a Bennett fracture subluxation. Most surgeons would aim to gain and hold adequate reduction of the fracture until bone union. This is harder to do nonoperatively but not impossible. In my experience use of a modified Bennett plaster holding the thumb MP joint flexed helps achieve and maintain reduction of the fracture in a plaster cast in most but not all cases. Thus many of these injuries can be treated nonoperatively and an adequate reduction achieved and maintained. In theory this should give as good an outcome as successful surgical treatment. Ultimately one or more RCTs comparing nonsurgical or surgical treatments are required to advance the treatment of this common injury.

Base of Middle Phalanx Injuries

Fractures of the base of the middle phalanx are difficult to treat. The two common injuries are dorsal fracture subluxations (dislocations) and pilon fractures. A wide range of treatments are available: from immobilization to dynamic external fixation, to immediate hemi-hamate arthroplasty.

Stable injuries, particularly fracture subluxations with a fracture of the base of the middle phalanx of less than one-third on the lateral radiograph or pilon fractures without too much displacement, seem to do well with nonoperative treatment.

Typically the remainder are treated surgically. With surgical treatment, although many patients achieve good results, there are some poor results especially if a postoperative infection occurs. Recent work suggests that lateral flexion radiographs, comparable with the lateral extension radiographs in the assessment of stability in bony mallet injuries, can predict the injuries that need surgery and those that do not. Patients attending their first outpatient clinic appointment within 10 days of injury, are encouraged to flex their injured finger as much as possible, ideally at least 40° at the PIP joint. A lateral flexion radiograph is performed. If this shows gliding (**Figs. 7** and **8**), specifically not pivoting, then the finger is treated with early mobilization anticipating a good outcome with little pain and a range of motion of at least 10° to 90°, as good as reported surgical series.

If the middle phalanx pivots about the volar margin of the bulk of the base of the middle phalanx as the finger flexes then there is likely to be a poor outcome and surgery is recommended (these patients often struggle to flex > 20°). It has not been ethical to treat the fingers that pivot, nonoperatively to assess whether surgery would have been needed. I have treated 10 fingers that glide with consistent results even when the fracture pattern, including an increased coronal width of the base of the middle phalanx (see **Fig. 8**), would suggest that surgery is required. I recommend careful and regular review for a minimum of 3 weeks from injury, with repeat radiographs to ensure there is no further late collapse of the fracture and to ensure that good early mobilization occurs. So far I have not seen late collapse or any poor outcomes.

CONSIDERATIONS IN DECIDING ON CONSERVATIVE TREATMENT

There are many problems with the published literature in the treatment of common hand fractures: there are few RCTs; there is bias in many of the

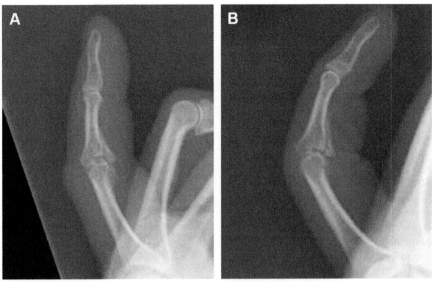

Fig. 7. (*A*) Pilon fracture at the PIP joint. (*B*) Pilon fracture gliding with flexion.

studies; often incomplete data; outdated outcome reporting; and in particular inadequate descriptions of the methods especially for nonoperative techniques. Although it is recognized that closed reduction and percutaneous K wiring is different from ORIF, papers often do not differentiate clearly between uninhibited mobilization, supervised mobilization with regular follow-up, and immobilization and follow-up. In addition the quality of postoperative care is rarely described despite its importance in assessing and maintaining fracture alignment in the first few weeks following injury.

The available data suggest that for the fractures described previously, surgery either does not reliably confer benefit over good nonoperative treatment or those requiring surgery can be selectively reduced especially by considering gliding or pivoting. For some injuries surgery is

rarely likely to be required (eg, spiral metacarpal fracture). For others although nonoperative treatment should usually be tried first, surgery is likely to be required often (eg, Bennett fractures). Because surgery typically costs more in patient risk and health care costs, it suggests that nonoperative treatment should be the default position for most of these injuries, accepting the need for clinical judgment for individual cases. That is the predominant clinical approach in the United Kingdom.

This review of the literature also highlights the dichotomies between authors recommending (at times vigorously) a range of different treatments for the same injuries. There are many possible reasons: surgeon preference or bias; a misunderstanding of the anatomy and pathology of the injury; an overemphasis on biomechanical or cadaveric studies that may not apply in clinical practice; an overemphasis on bone union that may not affect outcome; an overemphasis on anatomic reduction of intra-articular fractures that may not reliably affect outcome; and possibly most of all, the variability of the injuries such that a subgroup of each type of injury does poorly with one type of treatment, often nonoperative treatment, which skews the reported/perceived outcomes of that treatment. This subset bias requires closer observation/larger series to avoid mistreatment.

Research efforts should focus on areas where one might make a significant difference ahead of tackling those with marginal gains. Different patterns of displaced phalangeal fractures, and

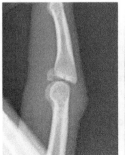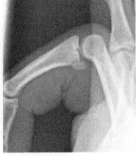

Fig. 8. PIP joint fracture subluxation gliding with flexion. PIP, proximal inter-phaangeal.

proximal interphalangeal joint fracture subluxations or pilon fractures, are two topics in hand fracture management where the optimal treatments are unclear and where research could make a considerable difference.

This is not a diatribe against surgical treatment of these fractures or against innovation. I look forward to new, probably less invasive techniques, such as intramedullary screw fixation,[20–22] and more reliable techniques that will improve the outcomes for patients. Until then the literature shows the outcomes of nonoperative treatment of most of these fractures is so good that there needs to be a strong argument for surgery to justify the risks and costs of surgery. This article highlights the need to identify the subgroups that do badly with nonoperative treatment (where they exist), such as through large cohort studies of nonoperative treatment or to identify new insights, such as the role of gliding or pivoting in bony mallet injuries (Giddins 2016) to clarify which injuries need surgery. In addition any future studies of these injuries that report an improvement in outcome with surgery should ideally be run as RCTs in comparison with vigilant and clearly described nonoperative treatment, because a cohort or case series of operative treatment is unlikely to improve on the published data.

SUMMARY

The outcome of nonoperative treatment of many hand fractures is so good that surgery is rarely required, such as for spiral or long oblique metacarpal fractures, metacarpal neck fractures, and bony collateral ligament avulsions of the thumb and finger MP joints.[78–84] Slight shortening and some dorsal angulation in the metacarpal bone and displacement at the proximal part of the metacarpal bone are always tolerable without loss of hand function. In other types of fractures there is a clear role for nonoperative treatment, such as for Bennett fractures and bony mallet injuries but also for surgical treatment. The aim should be to define the subgroups better to advise more reliably where surgery is likely to be beneficial and where it is not. Future novel techniques may change how clinicians treat these injuries.

REFERENCES

1. Diwaker HN, Stothard J. The role of internal fixation in closed fractures of the proximal phalanges and metacarpals in adults. J Hand Surg Br 1986;11: 103–8.
2. Barton N. Fractures of the hand. J Bone Joint Surg Br 1984;66:159–67.
3. AL-Qattan M. Metacarpal shaft fractures of the fingers: treatment with interosseous loop wire fixation and immediate postoperative finger mobilisation in a wrist splint. J Hand Surg Br 2006;31:377–82.
4. Al-Qattan M. The use of a combination of cerclage and unicortical unterosseous loop dental wires for long oblique/spiral metacarpal shaft fractures. J Hand Surg Eur 2008;33:728–31.
5. Al-Qattan M, Al-Lazzam A. Long oblique/spiral mid-shaft metacarpal fractures of the fingers: treatment with cerclage wire fixation and immediate post-operative finger mobilisation in a wrist splint. J Hand Surg Eur 2007;32:637–40.
6. Al-Qattan M. Outcome of conservative management of spiral/long oblique fractures of the metacarpal shaft of the fingers using a palmar wrist splint and immediate mobilisation of the fingers. J Hand Surg Eur 2008;33:723–7.
7. Khan A, Giddins GEB. The outcome of conservative treatment of spiral metacarpal fractures and biomechanical proof of the role of the intermetacarpal ligaments in stabilising these injuries. J Hand Surg Eur Vol 2015;40:59–62.
8. Low C, Wong Y, Wong H. A cadaver study of the effects of dorsal angulation and shortening of the metacarpal shaft on the extension and flexion force ratios of the index and little fingers. J Hand Surg Br 1995;20:609–13.
9. Meunier MJ, Hentzen E, Ryan M, et al. Predicted effects of metacarpal shortening on interosseous muscle function. J Hand Surg Am 2004;29:689–93.
10. Strauch RJ, Rosenwasser MP, Lunt JG. Metacarpal shaft fractures: the effect of shortening on the extensor tendon mechanism. J Hand Surg Am 1998;23:519–23.
11. Wills J, Crum J, McCabe R, et al. The effect of metacarpal shortening on digital flexion force. J Hand Surg Eur Vol 2013;38:667–72.
12. Stern PJ. Fractures of the metacarpals and phalanges. In: Green DP, Hotchkiss RN, Pederson WC, et al, editors. Green's operative hand surgery. 5th edition. New York: Elsevier, Churchill Livingstone; 2005. p. 277–341.
13. Ali A, Hamman J, Mass DP. The biomechanical effects of angulated boxer's fractures. J Hand Surg Am 1999;24:835–44.
14. Smith RJ, Peimer CA. Injuries to the metacarpal bones and joints. Adv Surg 1977;11:341–74.
15. Bloem JJAM. The treatment and prognosis of uncomplicated dislocated fractures of the metacarpals and phalanges. Arch Chir Neerl 1971;23:55–65.
16. Kilbourne BC, Paul EG. The use of small bone screws in the treatment of metacarpal, metatarsal, and phalangeal fracture. J Bone Joint Surg Am 1958;40:375–83.
17. Diao E, Welbourn JH. Extraarticular fractures of the metacarpals. In: Berger R, Weiss A, editors. Hand

surgery, vol. 1. New York: Lippincott Williams & Wilkins; 2004. p. 139–51.

18. Poolman RW, Goslings JC, Lee JB, et al. Conservative treatment for closed fifth (small finger) metacarpal neck fractures. Cochrane Database Syst Rev 2005;(3):CD003210.

19. Orbay JL, Touhami A. The treatment of unstable metacarpal and phalangeal shaft fractures with flexible nonlocking and locking intramedullary nails. Hand Clin 2006;22:279–86.

20. Borbas P, Dreu M, Poggetti A, et al. Treatment of proximal phalangeal fractures with an antegrade intramedullary screw: a cadaver study. J Hand Surg Eur Vol 2016;41:683–7.

21. del Piñal F, Moraleda E, Rúas JS, et al. Minimally invasive fixation of fractures of the phalanges and metacarpals with intramedullary cannulated headless compression screws. J Hand Surg Am 2015; 40:692–700.

22. Giesen T, Gazzola R, Poggetti A, et al. Intramedullary headless screw fixation for fractures of the proximal and middle phalanges in the digits of the hand: a review of 31 consecutive fractures. J Hand Surg Eur Vol 2016;41:688–94.

23. Downing ND, Davis TRC. Intramedullary fixation of unstable metacarpal fractures. Hand Clin 2006;22: 269–77.

24. Faraj AA, Davis TRC. Percutaneous intramedullary fixation of metacarpal shaft fractures. J Hand Surg Br 1999;24:76–9.

25. Foucher G. 'Bouquet' osteosynthesis in metacarpal neck fractures: a series of 66 patients. J Hand Surg Am 1995;20:86–90.

26. Margic K. External fixation of closed metacarpal and phalangeal fractures of digits. A prospective study of one hundred consecutive patients. J Hand Surg Br 2006;31:30–40.

27. Westbrook AP, Davis TR, Armstrong D, et al. The clinical significance of malunion of fractures of the neck and shaft of the little finger metacarpal. J Hand Surg Eur 2008;33:732–9.

28. Strub B, Schindele S, Sonderegger J, et al. Intramedullary splinting or conservative treatment for displaced fractures of the little finger metacarpal neck? A prospective study. J Hand Surg Eur Vol 2010;35:725–9.

29. Bekler H, Gokce A, Beyzadeoglu T. Avulsion fractures from the base of phalanges of the fingers. Tech Hand Up Extrem Surg 2006;10:157–61.

30. Bischoff R, Büchler U, De Roche R, et al. Clinical results of tension band fixation of avulsion fractures of the hand. J Hand Surg Am 1994;19: 1019–26.

31. Gee TC, Pho RWH. Avulsion-fracture at the proximal attachment of the radial collateral ligament of the fifth metacarpophalangeal joint: a case report. J Hand Surg Am 1982;7:526–7.

32. Gross DL, Moneim M. Radial collateral ligament avulsion fracture of the metacarpophalangeal joint in the small finger. Orthopaedics 1998;21:814–5.

33. Mikami Y, Takata H, Oishi K. Kirschner wire stabilization of collateral ligament avulsion fractures of the base of the proximal phalanx. J Hand Surg Eur Vol 2011;36:78–9.

34. Schubiner JM, Mass DP. Operation for collateral ligament ruptures of the metacarpophalangeal joints of the fingers. J Bone Joint Surg Br 1989;71:388–9.

35. Shewring DJ, Thomas RH. Avulsion fractures from the base of the proximal phalanges of the fingers. J Hand Surg Br 2003;28:10–4.

36. Sawant N, Kulikov Y, Giddins GEB. Outcome following conservative treatment of metacarpophalangeal collateral ligament avulsion fractures of the finger. J Hand Surg Eur Vol 2007;32:102–4.

37. Sorene ED, Goodwin DR. Non-operative treatment of displaced avulsion fractures of the ulnar base of the proximal phalanx of the thumb. Scand J Plast Reconstr Surg Hand Surg 2003;37:225–7.

38. Giele H, Martin J. The two-level ulnar collateral ligament injury of the metacarpophalangeal joint of the thumb. J Hand Surg Br 2003;28:92–3.

39. Dinowitz M, Trumble T, Hanel D, et al. Failure of cast immobilization for thumb ulnar collateral ligament avulsion fractures. J Hand Surg Am 1997;22:1057–63.

40. Kuz JE, Husband JB, Tokar N, et al. Outcome of avulsion fractures of the ulnar base of the proximal phalanx of the thumb treated nonsurgically. J Hand Surg Am 1999;24:275–82.

41. Kozin SH, Bishop AT. Tension wire fixation of avulsion fractures at the thumb metacarpophalangeal joint. J Hand Surg Am 1994;19:1027–31.

42. Edelstein DM, Kardashian G, Lee SK. Radial collateral ligament injuries of the thumb. J Hand Surg Am 2008;33:760–70.

43. Katz V, Loy S, Alnot JY. Sprains of the radial collateral ligament of the metacarpophalangeal joint of the thumb. A series of 14 cases. Ann Chir Main 1998;17:7–24.

44. Melone CP Jr, Beldner S, Basuk RS. Thumb collateral ligament injuries. An anatomic basis for treatment. Hand Clin 2000;16:345–57.

45. Smith RJ. Post-traumatic instability of the metacarpophalangeal joint of the thumb. J Bone Joint Surg Am 1997;59:14–21.

46. Camp RA, Weatherwax RJ, Miller EB. Chronic posttraumatic radial instability of the thumb metacarpophalangeal joint. J Hand Surg Am 1980;5:221–5.

47. Doty J, Rudd J, Jemison M. Radial collateral ligament injury of the thumb with a Stener-like lesion. Orthopedics 2010;33:959.

48. Köttstorfer J, Hofbauer M, Krusche-Mandl I, et al. Avulsion fracture and complete rupture of the thumb radial collateral ligament. Arch Orthop Trauma Surg 2013;133:583–8.

49. Auchingloss JM. Mallet-finger injuries: a prospective controlled trial of internal and external splintage. Hand 1982;14:168–73.

50. Badia A, Riano F. A simple fixation method for unstable bony mallet finger. J Hand Surg Am 2004;29:1051–5.

51. Bauze A, Bain GI. Internal suture for mallet finger fracture. J Hand Surg Br 1999;24:688.

52. Cheon SJ, Lim JM, Cha HS. Treatment of bony mallet finger using a modified pull-out wire suture technique. J Hand Surg Eur Vol 2011;36:247–9.

53. Damron TA, Engber WD. Surgical treatment of mallet finger fractures by tension band technique. Clin Orthop Relat Res 1994;(300):133–40.

54. Darder-Prats A, Fernández-García E, Fernández-Gabarda R, et al. Treatment of mallet finger fractures by the extension-block K-wire technique. J Hand Surg Br 1998;23:802–5.

55. Fritz D, Lutz M, Arora R, et al. Delayed single Kirschner wire compression technique for mallet fracture. J Hand Surg Br 2005;30:180–4.

56. Hiwatari R, Saito S, Shibayama M. The 'chased method' of mini screw fixation: a percutaneous surgical approach to treating mallet fractures. J Hand Surg Eur Vol 2012;39:784–6.

57. Ishiguro T, Itoh Y, Yabe Y, et al. Extension block with Kirschner wire for fracture dislocation of the distal interphalangeal joint. Tech Hand Up Extrem Surg 1997;1:95–102.

58. King HJ, Shin SJ, Kang ES. Complications of operative treatment for mallet fractures of the distal phalanx. J Hand Surg Br 2001;26:28–31.

59. Kronlage SC, Faust D. Open reduction and screw fixation of mallet fractures. J Hand Surg Br 2004;29:135–8.

60. Pegoli L, Toh S, Arai K, et al. The Ishiguro extension block technique for the treatment of mallet finger fracture: indications and clinical results. J Hand Surg Am 2003;28:15–7.

61. Rocchi L, Genitiempo M, Fanfani F. Percutaneous fixation of mallet fractures by the "umbrella handle" technique. J Hand Surg Br 2006;31:407–12.

62. Teoh LC, Lee JY. Mallet fractures: a novel approach to internal fixation using a hook plate. J Hand Surg Eur Vol 2007;32:24–30.

63. Stern PJ, Kastrup JJ. Complications and prognosis of treatment of mallet finger. J Hand Surg Am 1988;13:329–34.

64. Webhe MA, Schnieder LH. Mallet fractures. J Bone Joint Surg Am 1984;66:658–69.

65. Okafor B, Mbubaegbu C, Munshi I, et al. Mallet deformity of the finger. Five-year follow-up of conservative treatment. J Bone Joint Surg Br 1997;79:544–7.

66. Handoll HH, Vaghela MV. Interventions for treating mallet finger injuries [review]. Cochrane Database Syst Rev 2004;(3):CD004574.

67. Stark HH, Gainor BJ, Ashworth CR, et al. Operative treatment of intra-articular fractures of the dorsal aspect of the distal phalanx of digits. J Bone Joint Surg Am 1987;69:892–6.

68. Kim JK, Kim DJ. The risk factors associated with subluxation of the distal interphalangeal joint in mallet fracture. J Hand Surg Eur Vol 2015;40:63–7.

69. Giddins GE. Bony mallet finger injuries: assessment of stability with extension stress testing. J Hand Surg Eur Vol 2016;41:696–700.

70. Moradi A, Braun Y, Oflazoglu K, et al. Factors associated with subkuxation in mallet fracture. J Hand Surg Eur Vol 2017;42(2):176–81.

71. Edwards G, Giddins GE. Management of Bennett's fractures: a review of treatment outcomes. J Hand Surg Eur Vol 2017;42(2):201–3.

72. Livesley PJ. The conservative management of Bennett's fracture-dislocation: a 26-year follow-up. J Hand Surg Br 1990;15:291–4.

73. Leclère FM, Jenzer A, Husler R, et al. 7-year follow-up after open reduction and internal screw fixation in Bennett fractures. Arch Orthop Trauma Surg 2012;132:1045–51.

74. Cannon SR, Dowd GS, Williams DH, et al. A long-term study following Bennett's fracture. J Hand Surg Br 1986;11:426–31.

75. Griffiths JC. Fractures at the base of the first metacarpal bone. J Bone Joint Surg Br 1964;46:712–9.

76. Kjaer-Petersen K, Langhoff O, Andersen K. Bennett's fracture. J Hand Surg Br 1990;15:58–61.

77. Oosterbos CJ, de Boer HH. Non-operative treatment of Bennett's fracture: a 13 year follow up. J Orthop Trauma 1995;9:23–7.

78. Giddins GE. The non-operative management of hand fractures. J Hand Surg Eur Vol 2015;40:33–41.

79. Tang JB. Efficient and elaborate treatment of hand fractures. J Hand Surg Eur Vol 2015;40:7.

80. Gehrmann SV, Kaufmann RA, Grassmann JP, et al. Fracture-dislocations of the carpometacarpal joints of the ring and little finger. J Hand Surg Eur Vol 2015;40:84–7.

81. Tang JB, Blazar PE, Giddins G, et al. Overview of indications, preferred methods and technical tips for hand fractures from around the world. J Hand Surg Eur Vol 2015;40:88–97.

82. Wada T, Oda T. Mallet fingers with bone avulsion and DIP joint subluxation. J Hand Surg Eur Vol 2015;40:8–15.

83. Liverneaux PA, Ichihara S, Hendriks S, et al. Fractures and dislocation of the base of the thumb metacarpal. J Hand Surg Eur Vol 2015;40:42–50.

84. Neumeister MW, Webb K, McKenna K. Non-surgical management of metacarpal fractures. Clin Plast Surg 2014;41:451–61.

85. Landsman JC, Seitz WH Jr, Froimson AI, et al. Splint immobilization of gamekeeper's thumb. Orthopedics 1995;18:1161–5.

86. Hofmeister EP, Mazurek MT, Shin AY, et al. Extension block pinning for large mallet fractures. J Hand Surg Am 2003;28(3):453–9.

87. Takami H, Takahashi S, Ando M. Operative treatment of mallet finger due to intra-articular fracture of the distal phalanx. Arch Orthop Trauma Surg 2000; 120(1-2):9–13.

88. Tetik C, Gudemez E. Modification of the extension block Kirschner wire technique for mallet fractures. Clin Orthop Relat Res 2002;404:284–90.

Current European Practice in the Treatment of Proximal Interphalangeal Joint Arthritis

CrossMark

Daniel B. Herren, MD, MHA

KEYWORDS

- Arthroplasty • Proximal interphalangeal joint • Conservative treatment • Osteoarthritis • Finger joint
- Arthritis • Function

KEY POINTS

- Joint arthroplasty of the fingers is one of the options to treat painful destroyed proximal interphalangeal joints. It is gaining more and more popularity in Europe, especially in the growing population suffering from osteoarthritis of these joints.
- The most popular prostheses are Silastic implants, which provide predictable results with low revision rates. The main disadvantage is lateral instability, which can lead to significant joint deformity and the risk of implant breakage over time.
- Newer implants include 2-component hard bearing joints that mimic the joint constrain to maintain lateral stability and better correct deformity of finger joints.
- In Europe, most surgeons prefer uncemented prostheses, but implant fixation remains an issue; additionally, loosening and subsidence are often seen complications.
- The newest generation of proximal interphalangeal joint prosthesis in Europe has a modular structure, allowing optimal tensioning of the joint and surrounding tissues.

INTRODUCTION

Among the different treatment options in proximal interphalangeal (PIP) joint disease, arthroplasty has gained a lot of popularity in the last few years and undergone a remarkable evolution.[1] New implants, different surgical approaches, and different rehabilitation are part of the development in this field. The main indication for PIP arthroplasty is this degenerative joint disease (ie, osteoarthritis [OA]). The treatment of post-traumatic conditions seems to be stable or even decreasing over the last few years probably due to improved fracture management. Likewise, PIP arthroplasty in rheumatoid arthritis (RA) has become less frequent because of improved treatment of RA.

Some studies suggest that the finger joints are the most common site of osteoarthritis in the entire musculoskeletal system.[2] It has been shown that the cumulative incidence of finger joint osteoarthritis is generally higher in women, but the distribution over the different finger joints is the same in both sexes.

The growing number of patients affected by this disease, together with the increasing therapeutic possibilities, makes this probably one of the fastest growing patient population in hand surgery, especially for PIP joint arthroplasty.

Disclosure: The author receive royalties from KLS Martin Tuttlingen, Germany, for one of the devices mentioned in the article (CapFlex prosthesis).
Hand Surgery Department, Schulthess Klinik, Lenggahlde 2, Zurich 8008 CHE, Switzerland
E-mail address: daniel.herren@kws.ch

Hand Clin 33 (2017) 489–500
http://dx.doi.org/10.1016/j.hcl.2017.04.002

INDICATIONS AND TREATMENT

The main symptom in PIP joint osteoarthritis is pain. The degree of functional impairment in the PIP joint after OA depends on which joints are affected, the degree of stiffness, and the range of the residual arc of motion. Stability of the interphalangeal joints is an important issue, especially in the radial digits for strong pinch with the thumb. Patients with an erosive and inflammatory type of OA in these joints may have significant instability and deformity, which must be addressed when evaluating surgical treatment options. Another important issue for patients, especially women, is aesthetics.

Diagnosis

The diagnosis of OA of the PIP joint is based mainly on the clinical picture and confirmed by radiographs (**Fig. 1**).

The initial phase of disease is an inflammatory process that comes to a halt at a later stage.[3] This explains why many patients have fewer symptoms at the end stage of the disease than at the beginning. It is recognized that radiographs and

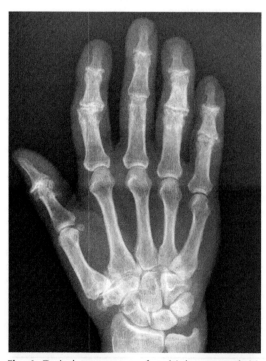

Fig. 1. Typical appearance of multiple osteoarthritis in the finger joints. Most often the DIP and PIP joints are involved, as well as the thumb saddle joint. The index PIP joint is often deviated to the ulnar side due to the mechanical forces in pinching with the thumb.

symptoms do not correlate. That is, the main reason that classifications and staging based on radiographs are rarely used. More important is the radiographic evaluation of the bone quality, namely defects and cyst formation. These and the presence of stiffness and deformity play a crucial role in the indication of possible surgical treatment options.

Conservative Treatment

Osteoarthritis is an incurable disease, and all attempts to treat this condition do no more than modify the symptoms. There is little evidence that any sort of prevention might be effective in stopping unaffected joints becoming part of the disease process. Besides oral medication, intra-articular treatment with an infliximab injection showed a good symptomatic benefit with a possible intra-articular disease-modifying action in erosive osteoarthritis of the hands[4] in a pilot study.

Conventional treatment includes analgesics and nonsteroidal anti-inflammatory drugs. Intra-articular viscosupplementation with hyaluronic acid has been shown to be effective in terms of pain relief and improved disability. Compared with intra-articular corticosteroids, it seems to have a longer benefit,[5] especially in the knee joint. However, personal experience does not support this observation for the finger joints.

Glucosamine and chondroitin are important components of the normal cartilage. Like viscosupplementation, the efficiency of glucosamine and chondroitin in the treatment of OA has been documented best in early arthritis in the knee joint.[6] They seem to reduce the need for anti-inflammatory drugs and improve functionality.[7] Because these substances show few adverse effects, many patients in Europe use these substances in the treatment of their finger arthritis, although there is no scientific evidence that they help.

Operative Treatment

Synovectomy
Surgical treatment options include synovectomy, joint replacement, and joint fusion. There is no conclusive literature on synovectomy of the PIP joint for OA. Synovectomy may be considered in the early stages of the osteoarthritic process when there is marked inflammation and the cartilage is still reasonably preserved.[8] Because no data on the mid- and long-term effects are available, the authors can only report their personal experience of this intervention. Overall, the results of this procedure are mixed at best.

Persistent, if not even exacerbated, pain and postoperative joint stiffness are possible complications. The authors have found that the best candidates for this procedure are patients who have had a good response to intra-articular steroid injections and have more than 80% cartilage preserved in the affected joints; this can, however, only be assessed intra-operatively. But even in this selected patient group, there is in the authors' experience only a 50-50 chance of a good result.

Joint fusion

The ideal goal for reconstruction of a disabled PIP joint is resolution of pain with functional mobility and adequate stability. The index and middle fingers are the pinching partners of the thumb, while the ulnar two fingers need mobility in order to grasp larger objects. Experience shows that pre-existing deformity and instability in the PIP joint are difficult to correct with a PIP arthroplasty, even with formal collateral ligament reconstruction and prolonged splinting during rehabilitation (**Fig. 2**). Arthrodesis should therefore be considered, especially in the radial digits, if lateral deformation of the PIP joint exceeds 30°. PIP joint fusion in a functionally good position provides adequate function, although fine

motor skills are affected. Woodworth and colleagues[9] evaluated the impact of simulated PIP joint fusion on all 4 fingers, with the PIP joints fixed in 40° of flexion. Low-demand activities of daily living suffered significantly when compared with unrestricted motion in all finger joints, while precision handling was perceived to be more difficult and required more compensation by the metacarpophalangeal (MP) joints.

Simultaneous fusions of the PIP and distal interphalangeal (DIP) joints in the same finger ray are possible, although precision handling will suffer. The combination of PIP arthroplasty and DIP fusion is functionally much better tolerated even if the range of motion in the PIP joint is limited.

For decades, joint fusion was the standard procedure for painful PIP joint destruction, and the functional results of this procedure were generally reported to be good.[10] Pellegrini and Burton[11] reviewed several patients who had undergone different procedures for PIP joint destruction. They observed that arthrodesis in the radial digits brought an improvement in the lateral pinch, while arthroplasty in the ulnar digits gave reasonable functional mobility with good pain relief. Based on this analysis, the authors were not able to make a definitive recommendation on the optimal procedure for destroyed PIP joints. Since that

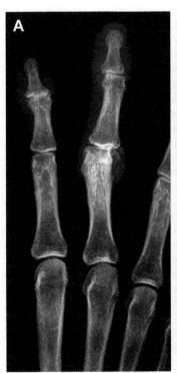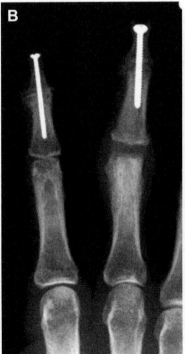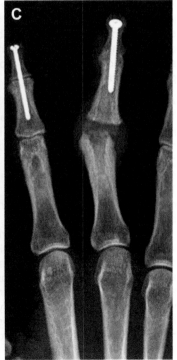

Fig. 2. (*A–C*) Silastic implant arthroplasty in a classic case of PIP osteoarthritis in combination with DIP arthrodesis. In the longer follow-up, there is a slight recurrence of the deviation.

publication, however, several authors have advocated the concept of reserving PIP arthroplasty for ulnar digits and treating the index finger, which is the main partner for pinching with the thumb, with PIP joint fusion.

Arthrodesis of the joint may be indicated in cases of severe instability and deformity of the PIP joint or joints with markedly damaged bone. Several techniques have been described for this procedure. Tension band wiring, plate fixation, and screw arthrodesis are the most common techniques. Tension band wiring has the advantage that compression of the arthrodesis site occurs during active motion. This technique is also cost-effective, using inexpensive hardware. The disadvantages are possible pin protrusion and painful hardware requiring subsequent metal removal.[10] Plate fixation, with screws usually 2.0 to 2.4 mm in size, allows rigid fixation at the desired angle and has gained a lot of popularity in Europe. It has the disadvantage of causing extensor tendon adhesions along the plate, thus limiting DIP motion. The newer-generation plates are so thin that hardware removal is not necessary in most patients. The screw fixation technique, preferably with a headless screw, is another option. Theoretically, a single screw has no rotational stability, but in practical use this does not cause any problems.[12] The main challenge with the screw technique is to achieve the desired fusion angle. This is not so easy to accomplish, especially for angles less than 30°. The straighter the fusion position, the more difficult it gets to obtain adequate purchase on the distal volar fragment. The screw also has more potential for protrusion on the proximal dorsal cortex.

Arthroplasty

There is a clear tendency to move away from PIP joint fusion toward arthroplasty. It is the understanding of an increasing number of hand surgeons, that even with a limited mobility a PIP arthroplasty gives better function than a fusion. Together with newer implants, which provide more lateral stability, the indication for PIP arthroplasty has increased in Europe.

Contraindications to PIP joint replacement include insufficient bone stock, missing or dysfunctional tendons and severe tendon imbalance, especially contracted boutonnière, and swan-neck deformities. In severely contracted joints with a long-standing history of immobility, PIP joint fusion in a functional position may be a better choice than implant arthroplasty. Severe joint instability and deformity of more than 30° are difficult to correct with an implant and area relative contraindications to arthroplasty.

Implants for the PIP Joint Arthroplasty

Choice of implants

The choice of implant and the approach used are the two most frequently discussed issues. A variety of implants is available, but only a few series with adequate long-term follow-up have been published. Silicone implants, introduced by Swanson in the late 1960s, are still the gold standard for newer generations of implants with respect to functional performance, revision rate, and long-term outcomes.[13] Silicone joint spacers carry a risk of implant breakage with instability and rarely silicone synovitis. Newer resurfacing type designs have become popular but have particular risks of dislocation and implant loosening.[14] Overall, the silicone spacer produces consistent results with good pain relief and reasonable function, with a range of motion between 40° and 60° active flexion/extension. Only a few cases of silicone synovitis have been reported, and, although implant failure is seen, it does not necessarily lead to revision.[15–18]

There is a newer generation of silicone implants such as the NewFlex (Stryker, MI, USA) prosthesis.[19] These devices have a more rectangular shape, which should provide better stability of the joint. Because the anatomic shape of the subcapital bone of the proximal phalanx is more elliptical, the rectangular shape of these hinges may interfere to some extent with the extensor mechanism, so it is felt to be essential that the implant is placed correctly. No randomized controlled trials with series of different silicone implants in the PIP joint are available; analysis of the different case series suggests similar results for most of the silicone implant designs.[20]

The newest generation of PIP joint prostheses follows the principles of surface replacement with a 2-component concept. The proximal component replaces the bicondylar head of the proximal phalanx, and the distal component has some sort of a cup, which articulates with the head. However, most do not represent a real resurfacing concept, because a significant amount of bone has to be resected; additionally, long stems for both components are needed to provide adequate fixation.

Several material combinations are available, from the classic chrome cobalt/polyethylene to ceramic/ceramic and pyrocarbon/pyrocarbon. Most of these implants can be used without cement, although some of them require cementing for primary fixation in the bone. Most surgeons in Europe prefer uncemented implants, because revision is easier; additionally, removal of the implant causes less damage and bone loss.

Overall, the newer generation of PIP implants based on resurfacing with more limited bone resection seems a logical development in PIP arthroplasty, but most of them have not yet stood the test of time; real-life long-term follow-up series are still lacking for most implant designs.

The choice of implant depends on several factors, including the surgeon's experience, the local anatomy, especially the bone stock, and the surgical approach. Silicone devices, which act as joint spacers, are by far the most forgiving implants. They provide reproducible results even in cases with limited bone stock and in surgeons with limited surgical experience. They can be implanted easily using different surgical approaches. More complex, 2-component joints need adequate bone stock, with no large cystic defects, as they are uncemented implants. Correct placement, with the goal of restoring the biomechanical center of rotation, needs some experience. Some of these implants are supplied with resection guides, which can be used only with a dorsal approach. In addition, some prostheses need more space for implantation, which also means that a dorsal or lateral approach is required.

Surgical approach

Different surgical approaches have been described to implant PIP joint replacements.[21] All of them have theoretic advantages and disadvantages. So far, no single approach has proved to be superior to the others, although the theoretic advantages of the volar approach are now being popularized.

The dorsal approach is the most widely used and technically least demanding in comparison with the volar and lateral approaches. It is also required when certain soft tissue conditions, such as mild swan neck or boutonnière deformity, are to be corrected at the same time. A straight or slightly curved longitudinal incision is performed. The dorsal veins should be preserved if possible and care taken with the dorsal nerve branch to the PIP joint. Several techniques have been described to access the joint. Swanson[18] advocated a midline split of the central slip of the extensor tendon. Some surgeons believe that care should be taken to preserve the central part of the central slip. It should be mobilized so that a good view of the joint is possible. If it is released together with the joint capsule, it can be easily reattached, but that may not be necessary. Although Swanson insisted on a good refixation of the central slip, surgeons have moved away from transosseous reinsertion. It may compromise the gliding of the lateral bands and thus limits DIP joint mobility.

A possible alternative is the approach described by Chamay.[22] He used a V-shaped extensor flap, which offers a good view of the joint and allows a long stable suture line for tendon closure. It has lost its popularity due to several, unfortunately unpublished, reports of complications with it. The authors have also moved away from this technique, because they have seen some significant tendon calcifications and in several patients a hyperextension deformity that develops over time.

After exposing the joint, the most dorsal parts of the 2 collateral ligaments are released; this gives full access to the joint with a good overview. Dorsal and volar osteophytes can now be removed if needed. The volar osteophyte is functionally more important than the dorsal osteophyte, because it may inhibit flexion, while the dorsal bone proliferation typically has no impact on the joint mobility. The bone is prepared according to the needs of the selected implant. For silicone implants, the resection line is planed according to the implant size (most often size 1 in the original Swanson design), and care should be taken to preserve as much of the collateral ligaments as possible. After bone preparation, the trial implant is inserted, and a trial reduction is performed. The tension should be chosen so that full flexion and, in particular, extension are possible. Either a smaller implant or more bone resection is needed if there is an extensor lag. In 2-component implants, the additional resection should be made on the distal side, which provides a better reconstruction of the natural center of rotation of the joint. When there is significant joint deformity or deficient collateral ligaments, a reinforcement suture of the ligaments and/or a staged release can be applied on the contracted side. The sutures are passed within the ligament and reinserted through drill holes in the proximal phalanx.

The joint should now be well balanced but with a full passive range of motion still being possible. Overtight collateral ligament reconstruction needs to be avoided, because it may provoke excessive scarring and thus stiffness. The authors tend to leave the joint supple, because overtensioning often produces pain.

Postoperatively, it is virtually impossible to correct any deformity remaining on the operating table, even with a careful rehabilitation program. Collateral ligament reconstruction should be considered carefully, because extended soft tissue reconstruction around a PIP implant tends to produce a stiff joint. If the joint has gross instability, arthrodesis might be the better option.

The volar approach has, at least theoretically, several advantages over other approaches.[23] The tendons are not violated with this technique, and, in particular, the delicate extensor mechanism remains untouched. The venous drainage is less compromised, which results in less postoperative swelling and easier subsequent rehabilitation. However, the volar approach is technically more demanding and offers less space for the implantation of an artificial joint. In addition, pre-existing tendon imbalances are more difficult to correct. The technique described by Simmen offers good access to the joint.[15] A Bruner incision forms a radially based skin flap. The 2 neurovascular bundles are identified and protected. The ulnar bundle has to be mobilized, while the radial bundle remains with the skin flap. The flexor tendon sheath is opened transversely in the area of the A3 pulley on both the volar and the dorsal sides. On the ulnar and the radial sides, the incision is continued to form a sleeve, which includes the release of the accessory collateral ligaments (**Fig. 3**). Access to the joint is now

achieved with hyperextension. Some release of the ulnar collateral ligament may be needed if the joint is not supple enough to get a good exposure. The osteophytes, especially those on the volar side, can now be removed. This is important, because they may be a potential site of impingement with the implant in flexion. The head of the proximal phalanx can now be resected, but care has to be taken to identify the ulnar neurovascular bundle and protect it with retractors. Preparation of the bone and implantation of the prosthesis follow the same principles as for the dorsal approach.

For closure, the pulley sleeve is retracted and reattached in its anatomic position. In cases with pre-existing deviation of the flexor tendon due to lateral deformity, tenolysis can help centralize the tendons. If needed, the collateral ligaments can be reinforced with sutures. It is important to test the passive range of motion again before final

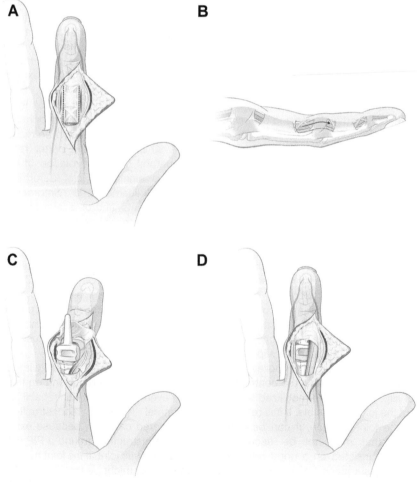

Fig. 3. Volar approach for PIP arthroplasty. Through a Bruner incision, the pulley system is exposed and a sleeve formed including the volar plate and the accessory collateral ligaments. The joint can be exposed through hyperextension.

closure. The rehabilitation program follows the principles outlined for the dorsal approach, but no special protection of the extensor tendons is needed; even passive motion is allowed.

The lateral approach is the least common approach used for PIP implants.[24] The incision goes along the midline, typically on the ulnar side of the finger and curves dorsally on the middle phalanx. After releasing the oblique and transverse fibers of the retinacular ligaments, the extensor apparatus is elevated and can be mobilized laterally, with the insertion of the central slip remaining intact. The ulnar neurovascular bundle remains on the volar side of the joint. The ulnar collateral ligament has to be detached completely in such a way that the joint can be opened on the radial side. This is best done with a triangular proximally based flap that can be reflected proximally. The implant can be inserted as described previously. For closure, it is essential to reattach the ulnar collateral ligament in such a way that active rehabilitation is possible. The ulnar side has to be protected with buddy splinting for up to 6 weeks.

Rehabilitation

Rehabilitation must be individualized according to the intra-operative stability, the collateral ligament status, and the scarring behavior of the patient. Although some authors still choose their rehabilitation program according to the implant used and the surgical approach, it appears that the concept of individualization is more important. The criteria are: bone quality, implant type, pre-existing and residual joint deformity, and soft tissue quality.

Resting splints in the intrinsic plus position are worn for up to 6 weeks. Buddy splinting to the neighboring radial finger, with a figure of eight dressing, is a good way of protecting the collateral ligaments and yet still allowing active and passive motion. Individual adaptations need to be made during the rehabilitation program. If the joints become stiff early, more vigorous mobilization is needed. In general, dynamic splinting is rarely needed and often not tolerated by the soft tissues until 4 to 6 weeks after surgery. Regardless of the surgical approach, an extensor lag is the most commonly observed deficit. Although functionally often not very limiting, patients do not like it if it exceeds about 30°. Interestingly enough, it is observed in all different approaches. In the volar approach, the scarring of the volar plate and the flexor tendon sheath is responsible. On the dorsal side, the extensor tendon healing with subsequent loss of free gliding or a certain excess length of the extensor mechanism may be the reason for the loss of extension. In addition, the collateral ligaments tend to shorten in the healing process and add to the restriction of extension.

Night splints in extension and dynamic extensor splints may help to correct this deficit.

OUTCOMES

Overall, the results of PIP joint arthroplasty are reasonably uniform. Pain relief is good to excellent, and the mean range of motion for almost all implants, including the newer designs, is 40° to 60°; there is a high recurrence of pre-existing deformities in Silastic implants but good potential for correction in 2-component prostheses.[25] In most series, the PIP joint range of motion does not improve appreciably, and there is no clear correlation between preoperative mobility and postoperative range of motion.[15] The newer designs do not improve the active range of motion; moreover, they have a greater potential for complications compared with silicone implants.[26,27]

COMMONLY USED IMPLANTS IN EUROPE

Although no statistical reports are available, it seems that silicone implants are still the most widely used prostheses for PIP joint replacement in Europe. Despite the unfavorable reports about pyrolytic carbon implants, they are still in use. The series of Reissner and colleagues[14] from 2014 summarizes the results of this implant well. In a 10 year follow-up study, there were moderate clinical results with a mean range of motion of 40° and a high rate of implant migration rate. Pain relief was significant, with a reduction from a preoperative pain scale (VAS) of 7.6 to 0.7 postoperatively. The results seemed to be stable over time. Another European study is the series of Meier and colleagues.[28] In 20 patients, an 80% satisfaction rate was found. Two implants had to be removed

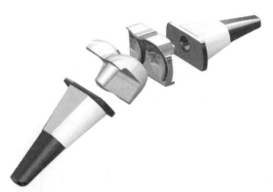

Fig. 4. The Tactys (Stryker) implant. A modular PIP prosthesis with a polyethlyen/metallic combination with interchangeable parts for full modularity. The stems are hydroxyapatite coated for cement-free implantation. (*Courtesy of* Stryker, Pusignan, France; with permission.)

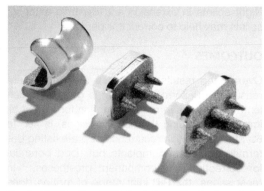

Fig. 5. The CapFlex (KLS Martin) prosthesis. A modular resurfacing prosthesis with a polyethlyen/metal combination. The different heights of the polyethylene allows optimal tensioning of the joints collateral ligaments. (*Courtesy of* KLS Martin, Tuttlingen, Germany; with permission.)

due to dislocation. Implant migration was found in 9 prosthetic components; none had to be revised. The mean range of motion was 50°.

A newer implant development from Europe is the Tactys prosthesis (Johnson&Johnson, NJ, USA) (**Fig. 4**). In 2016, Athlani and colleagues[29] published the first series of this implant with a minimum follow-up of 2 years. All implants, which were all operated through a dorsal approach, were still in place at follow-up, with no signs of loosening. The 4 patients who needed reoperation had to be treated mainly due to tendon adhesions. The range of motion increased from a mean of 39° preoperatively to 58° postoperatively. Pain decreased on the VAS from 6.5 to 1.9.

A real surface replacement arthroplasty has also been developed; the CapFlex prosthesis (KLS Martin Tuttlingen, Germany). It is an uncemented implant with short stem fixation and a modular polyethylene inlay. The different inlay thickness allows for collateral ligament tensioning (**Fig. 5**). The first case series of this implant was published in 2015.[25] In a prospective study, 10 PIP joints, implanted with a dorsal Chamay approach, were followed for at least 1 year (**Fig. 6**). All implants showed good osteointegration and no signs of loosening. The mean preoperative range of motion was 42°; this increased to 51° postoperatively. Two joints had to be reoperated due to extensor tendon adhesion and consequent stiffness.

Table 1 summarizes the results of different implant arthroplasty for the PIP joint.[11,13,15–17,20,25,28–38]

COMPLICATIONS OF PROXIMAL INTERPHALANGEAL ARTHROPLASTY

The complication rate in PIP arthroplasty is significant. Although the main problems of silicone devices are implant failure and cystic bone formation with time,[16] more complex joints might show implant loosening and joint dislocation. In the long-term follow-up, it is to be expected that 10% to 30% of the silicone implants at the PIP level will fracture (**Fig. 7**). This is clearly less than

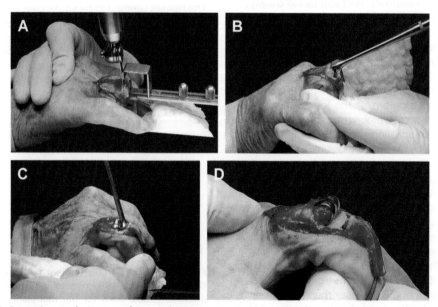

Fig. 6. (*A*) Operation technique surface replacement: resection guide for precise bone preparation. Dorsal approach with a Chamay tendon flap. (*B*) Modulator, which forms the bone to exact fit of the implant. (*C*) Distal preparation of the fixation with proximal trail implant in situ. (*D*) Final implant setting.

Table 1
Summary of different published series on proximal interphalangeal implant arthroplasty

Author, Year	Type of Implant	Number of Implants	Follow-up	VAS Pain	Rom Pre/Post	Approach	Complications
Swanson,[30] 1972	Silicone	148	—	Satisfactory	—	—	—
Iselin & Pradet,[31] 1984	Silicone	222	—	66% = 0	—	—	—
Pellegrini & Burton,[11] 1990	Silicone	24	45	Satisfactory	56° post	Dorsal	35% periprosthetic osteolysis
Iselin et al,[17] 1995	Silicone	238	24	67% = 0	50° post	—	—
Lin, 1995	Silicone	69	40	97% = 0	44°/46°	Volar	7% implant fractures
Ashworth et al,[32] 1997	Silicone	99	68	67% = 0	38°/29°	—	10% implant fractures; 12% osteolysis
Herren & Simmen,[15] 2000	Silicone	59	28	81% = 0	59° post	Volar	—
Takigawa et al,[16] 2004	Silicone	70	78	1.2	26°/30°	Dorsal/volar	16% implant fractures
Bales et al,[13] 2014	Silicone	58	120	0.4	55°/50°	—	5% painful fractures
Herren et al,[33] 2006	Pyrocarbon	17	20.5	7.6/1.3	34°/42	Dorsal	47% implant subsidience
Meier et al,[28] 2007	Pyrocarbon	24	15	6.3/0.9	50°/—	Dorsal	37% implant subsidience
Chung et al,[40] 2009	Pyrocarbon	21	12	6.6/2.2	—	Dorsal	14% implant dislocations
Sweets & Stern,[34] 2011	Pyrocarbon	31	55	3 post	57°/31°	Dorsal	48% subsidience; 16% dislocation
Watts et al,[35] 2012	Pyrocarbon	97	60	—	25°/30°	Dorsal	7% implant dislocation; 4% subsidience
McGuire et al,[36] 2012	Pyrocarbon	57	27	Sig.improvement	30°/66°	Dorsal	40% implant subsidience
Reissner et al,[14] 2014	Pyrocarbon	15	115	7.6/0.7	36°/29°	Dorsal	Stable over time
Linscheid et al,[37] 1997	Cobalt-Chrome	66	54	improvement	35°/47°	Dorsal/volar	0.7% loosening (1 implant)
Jennings, 2008	SR-PIP	43	37	77% improvement	57°/58°	Dorsal/volar	26% revisions
Schindele et al,[25] 2015	CapFlex	10	12	100% improvement	42°/51°	Dorsal	20% soft tissue revisions
Jennings & Livingstone,[38] 2015	SR-PIP	39	111	77% improvement	57°/56°	Dorsal/volar	26% revisions
Athlani et al,[29] 2016	Tactys	22	33.5	6.5/1.0	40°/58°	Dorsal	27% periprosthetic ossification

Abbreviation: Rom, range of motion.

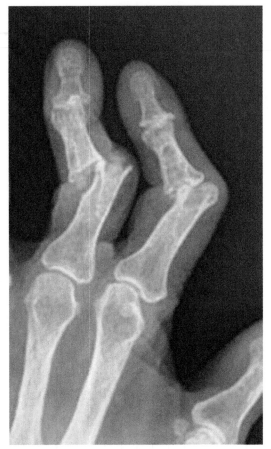

Fig. 7. Joint dislocation of broken Silastic implants with instability and massive deviation.

in the MCP joints, and these fractures do not always require revision surgery. In comparison with the MCP joint, the rate of silicone synovitis is less, and in the author's experience, only a few cases need revision for this problem. As already mentioned, recurrence of pre-existing deformity is high. The overall revision rate in the literature varies from 2% up to 13%.[13,15,16,24] In the series of 612 consecutive PIP silicone arthroplasties of the author and the colleagues over 10 years, with the majority of cases operated on for OA, there was a revision rate of 5.5%.[39] The main reasons for revision were pain, limited range of motion, and joint deformity, mainly ulnar deviation. Most patients showed a combination of these problems.

The most disabling complication is a hyperextension deformity after PIP arthroplasty. It should be avoided by all means, since it leaves a substantial functional deficit. It is more often seen with 2-component prostheses implanted via a dorsal approach. Reattachment of the central slip is to be avoided, since, together with an insufficient volar plate or a too loose implant, it limits flexion

of the PIP joint. Early dorsal block splinting may help to avoid this deformity.

The newer generation of prostheses, including pyrocarbon, ceramic, and other resurfacing implants, shows a relatively high complication rate with implant dislocation and problems with bone fixation in uncemented devices.[27,33,40,41] A permanent squeaking, unrelated to pain, has been seen with some of the implants. Overall the main reason for revision is the presence of soft tissue complications. Tendon scarring with stiffness and instability due to insufficient ligaments are the leading causes for reoperations. This is the reason that different authors call the PIP arthroplasty primarily a soft tissue procedure.

Hemi-hamate autograft arthroplasty is increasingly used in some regions of the world. Some European surgeons use this method.[42,43] In recent literature, a number of surgeons from Europe reported mechanical analysis of implant failure mechanism, and mid- to long-term outcomes after a certain type of implants to the PIP joint.[44–48]

REVISION OF PROXIMAL INTERPHALANGEAL ARTHROPLASTY

PIP arthroplasty revision remains a challenge with a high incidence of complications. Wagner and colleagues[49] found a lower rate of implant failure after revisions in Silastic and metal and polyethylene compared with pyrocarbon implants. Pain relief was good after revisions but often at the expense of a reduced range of motion. The authors published a series of silicone revision arthroplasties in 2014.[50] Revision surgery was most successful to treat severe stiffness and painful joints. Joint deformity, especially ulnar deviation, was difficult to correct.

SUMMARY

There is an increasing number of PIP arthroplasties performed in Europe. Most surgeons prefer meanwhile arthroplasty over arthrodesis even in radial fingers. Silastic arthroplasties are still the most widely used implants and provide consistent results with low revision rates even in long-term follow-up. The main disadvantage of the Silastic implants is the limited stability they provide, especially in counteracting lateral forces. Thus correction of pre-existing deformation is difficult. Soft tissue handling and postoperative scarring have a main influence on the results of PIP arthroplasty, regardless of the implant. Different surgical approaches are possible and have their advantages and disadvantages. The most popular approach in Europe is dorsal, but an increasing number of surgeons are trying the volar approach. Different surface replacement implants are on the market in Europe. Most surgeons use them as uncemented devices. The main advantage of these implants is the lateral stability provided through their more anatomic form. Revision of a failed PIP arthroplasty remains a challenge. Good indications are pain and stiffness. Correction of a deformity through a revision implant is less successful. Joint fusion, almost always requiring a bone graft, is often a better solution than revision arthroplasty for the radial 2 fingers.

REFERENCES

1. Kolling C, Herren DB, Simmen BR, et al. Changes in surgical intervention patterns in rheumatoid arthritis over 10 years in one centre. Ann Rheum Dis 2009; 68:1372–3.
2. Kalichman L, Cohen Z, Kobyliansky E, et al. Patterns of joint distribution in hand osteoarthritis: contribution of age, sex, and handedness. Am J Human Biol 2004;16:125–34.
3. Varju G, Pieper CF, Renner JB, et al. Assessment of hand osteoarthritis: correlation between thermographic and radiographic methods. Rheumatology (Oxford) 2004;43:915–9.
4. Fioravanti A, Fabbroni M, Cerase A, et al. Treatment of erosive osteoarthritis of the hands by intra-articular infliximab injections: a pilot study. Rheumatol Int 2009;29:961–5.
5. Strauss EJ, Hart JA, Miller MD, et al. Hyaluronic acid viscosupplementation and osteoarthritis: current uses and future directions. Am J Sports Med 2009; 37:1636–44.
6. Huskisson EC. Glucosamine and chondroitin for osteoarthritis. J Int Med Res 2008;36:1161–79.
7. Uebelhart D. Clinical review of chondroitin sulfate in osteoarthritis. Osteoarthritis Cartilage 2008; 16(Suppl 3):S19–21.
8. Gschwend N, Raemy H, Nittner H, et al. Long-term results of endoprosthetic joint replacement and synovectomy. Handchir Mikrochir Plast Chir 1986;18:135–49 [in German].
9. Woodworth JA, McCullough MB, Grosland NM, et al. Impact of simulated proximal interphalangeal arthrodeses of all fingers on hand function. J Hand Surg Am 2006;31:940–6.
10. Uhl RL. Proximal interphalangeal joint arthrodesis using the tension band technique. J Hand Surg Am 2007;32:914–7.
11. Pellegrini VD Jr, Burton RI. Osteoarthritis of the proximal interphalangeal joint of the hand: arthroplasty or fusion? J Hand Surg Am 1990;15:194–209.
12. Ayres JR, Goldstrohm GL, Miller GJ, et al. Proximal interphalangeal joint arthrodesis with the Herbert screw. J Hand Surg Am 1988;13:600–3.
13. Bales JG, Wall LB, Stern PJ. Long-term results of swanson silicone arthroplasty for proximal interphalangeal joint osteoarthritis. J Hand Surg Am 2014;39:455–61.
14. Reissner L, Schindele S, Hensler S, et al. Ten year follow-up of pyrocarbon implants for proximal interphalangeal joint replacement. J Hand Surg Eur Vol 2014;39:582–6.
15. Herren DB, Simmen BR. Palmar approach in flexible implant arthroplasty of the proximal interphalangeal joint. Clin Orthop Relat Res 2000;371:131–5.
16. Takigawa S, Meletiou S, Sauerbier M, et al. Long-term assessment of Swanson implant arthroplasty in the proximal interphalangeal joint of the hand. J Hand Surg Am 2004;29:785–95.
17. Iselin F, Conti E, Perrotte R, et al. Long-term results of proximal interphalangeal resection-arthroplasty using the Swanson Silastic implant. Ann Chir Main Memb Super 1995;14:126–33 [in French].
18. Swanson AB, de Groot Swanson G. Flexible implant resection arthroplasty of the proximal interphalangeal joint. Hand Clin 1994;10:261–6.
19. Namdari S, Weiss AP. Anatomically neutral silicone small joint arthroplasty for osteoarthritis. J Hand Surg Am 2009;34:292–300.
20. Stahlenbrecher A, Hoch J. Proximal interphalangeal joint silicone arthroplasty–comparison of Swanson and NeuFlex implants using a new evaluation score. Handchir Mikrochir Plast Chir 2009;41:156–65 [in German].
21. Cheah AE, Yao J. Surgical approaches to the proximal interphalangeal joint. J Hand Surg Am 2016; 41:294–305.
22. Chamay A. A distally based dorsal and triangular tendinous flap for direct access to the proximal interphalangeal joint. Ann Chir Main 1988;7:179–83.
23. Bouacida S, Lazerges C, Coulet B, et al. Proximal interphalangeal joint arthroplasty with Neuflex(R) implants: relevance of the volar approach and early rehabilitation. Chir Main 2014;33:350–5.
24. Merle M, Villani F, Lallemand B, et al. Proximal interphalangeal joint arthroplasty with silicone implants (NeuFlex) by a lateral approach: a series of 51 cases. J Hand Surg Eur Vol 2012;37:50–5.
25. Schindele SF, Hensler S, Audige L, et al. A modular surface gliding implant (CapFlex-PIP) for proximal interphalangeal joint osteoarthritis: a prospective case series. J Hand Surg Am 2015;40:334–40.
26. Stoecklein HH, Garg R, Wolfe SW. Surface replacement arthroplasty of the proximal interphalangeal joint using a volar approach: case series. J Hand Surg Am 2011;36:1015–21.
27. Wijk U, Wollmark M, Kopylov P, et al. Outcomes of proximal interphalangeal joint pyrocarbon implants. J Hand Surg Am 2010;35:38–43.
28. Meier R, Schulz M, Krimmer H, et al. Proximal interphalangeal joint replacement with pyrolytic

carbon prostheses. Oper Orthop Traumatol 2007;
19:1–15.

29. Athlani L, Gaisne E, Bellemere P. Arthroplasty of the proximal interphalangeal joint with the TACTYS(R) prosthesis: Preliminary results after a minimum follow-up of 2 years. Hand Surg Rehabil 2016;35: 168–78.

30. Swanson AB. Flexible implant resection arthroplasty. Hand 1972;4:119–34.

31. Iselin F, Pradet G. Resection arthroplasty with Swanson's implant for posttraumatic stiffness of proximal interphalangeal joints. Bull Hosp Jt Dis Orthop Inst 1984;44:233–47.

32. Ashworth CR, Hansraj KK, Todd AO, et al. Swanson proximal interphalangeal joint arthroplasty in patients with rheumatoid arthritis. Clin Orthop Relat Res 1997;342:34–7.

33. Herren DB, Schindele S, Goldhahn J, et al. Problematic bone fixation with pyrocarbon implants in proximal interphalangeal joint replacement: short-term results. J Hand Surg Br 2006;31:643–51.

34. Sweets TM, Stern PJ. Pyrolytic carbon resurfacing arthroplasty for osteoarthritis of the proximal interphalangeal joint of the finger. J Bone Joint Surg Am 2011;93:1417–25.

35. Watts AC, Hearnden AJ, Trail IA, et al. Pyrocarbon proximal interphalangeal joint arthroplasty: minimum two-year follow-up. J Hand Surg Am 2012;37:882–8.

36. McGuire DT, White CD, Carter SL, et al. Pyrocarbon proximal interphalangeal joint arthroplasty: outcomes of a cohort study. J Hand Surg Eur Vol 2012;37:490–6.

37. Linscheid RL, Murray PM, Vidal MA, et al. Development of a surface replacement arthroplasty for proximal interphalangeal joints. J Hand Surg Am 1997; 22:286–98.

38. Jennings CD, Livingstone DP. Surface replacement arthroplasty of the proximal interphalangeal joint using the SR PIP implant: long-term results. J Hand Surg Am 2015;40:469–73.e6.

39. Schindele S, Keuchel T, Herren DB. Revision arthroplasty of the PIP joint after primary failure of a Silicone implant. 16th Federation of the European Societies for Surgery of the Hand (FESSH) Meeting. Oslo (Norway), May 26–28, 2011.

40. Chung KC, Ram AN, Shauver MJ. Outcomes of pyrolytic carbon arthroplasty for the proximal interphalangeal joint. Plast Reconstr Surg 2009;123:1521–32.

41. Drake ML, Segalman KA. Complications of small joint arthroplasty. Hand Clin 2010;26:205–12.

42. Frueh FS, Calcagni M, Lindenblatt N. The hemihamate autograft arthroplasty in proximal interphalangeal joint reconstruction: a systematic review. J Hand Surg Eur Vol 2015;40:24–32.

43. Liodaki E, Xing SG, Mailaender P, et al. Management of difficult intra-articular fractures or fracture dislocations of the proximal interphalangeal joint. J Hand Surg Eur Vol 2015;40:16–23.

44. Drayton P, Morgan BW, Davies MC, et al. A biomechanical study of the effects of simulated ulnar deviation on silicone finger joint implant failure. J Hand Surg Eur Vol 2016;41:944–7.

45. Storey PA, Goddard M, Clegg C, et al. Pyrocarbon proximal interphalangeal joint arthroplasty: a medium to long term follow-up of a single surgeon series. J Hand Surg Eur Vol 2015;40:952–6.

46. Flannery O, Harley O, Badge R, et al. MatOrtho proximal interphalangeal joint arthroplasty: minimum 2-year follow-up. J Hand Surg Eur Vol 2016;41:910–6.

47. Proubasta IR, Lamas CG, Natera L, et al. Silicone proximal interphalangeal joint arthroplasty for primary osteoarthritis using a volar approach. J Hand Surg Am 2014;39:1075–81.

48. Tägil M, Geijer M, Abramo A, et al. Ten years' experience with a pyrocarbon prosthesis replacing the proximal interphalangeal joint. A prospective clinical and radiographic follow-up. J Hand Surg Eur Vol 2014;39:587–95.

49. Wagner ER, Luo TD, Houdek MT, et al. Revision proximal interphalangeal arthroplasty: an outcome analysis of 75 consecutive cases. J Hand Surg Am 2015;40:1949–55.e1.

50. Herren DB, Keuchel T, Marks M, et al. Revision arthroplasty for failed silicone proximal interphalangeal joint arthroplasty: indications and 8-year results. J Hand Surg Am 2014;39:462–6.

Treatment of Scaphoid Fractures
European Approaches

Joseph Dias, MD, FRCS, MBBS*,
Shanjitha Kantharuban, MBBCh, MRCS

KEYWORDS

- Scaphoid • Fracture • Europe • Treatment

KEY POINTS

- Scaphoid fractures account for 2% of all fractures, and in Europe, the incidence is 12.4/100,000/y. This article focuses on the current European perspective on the understanding and management of these injuries.
- Scaphoid fractures may be immobilized in cast or surgically fixed. Cast immobilization is still the treatment of choice in occult or stable fractures with 90% to 95% healing.
- Rates of union for nonoperative and operative management of undisplaced fractures are greater than 90%.
- Displaced fractures have a higher risk of nonunion. These fractures may benefit from reduction of the fracture fragments by closed, open, or arthroscopic methods and then internal fixation using headless compression screw or cannulated screw systems.

INTRODUCTION

In this article we present the current European perspective on the understanding and management of scaphoid injuries. Scaphoid fractures account for 2% of all fractures; it is the most commonly injured carpal bone, accounting for 90% of all carpal fractures.[1] In Europe, the reported incidence varies and ranges between 22 to 43 fractures in every 100,000 inhabitants,[2–4] but a recent study shows an incidence of 12.4 per 100,000 per year.[5] These fractures tend to occur in young and active patients, many of whom are dependent on the integrity of upper limb function for work and sport.[6]

ANATOMY

The scaphoid is an obliquely orientated bone situated on the radial aspect of the wrist joint. It is the only bone that spans both carpal rows. It is divided into 3 regions: proximal pole, waist, and distal pole. It has 6 surfaces, 3 of which are articular. The blood supply is mainly (75%) from branches of the radial artery that pass through the capsular attachment to the dorsal ridge and these also supply the proximal pole. The distal pole of the scaphoid has a reliable direct blood supply but the proximal pole is mostly supplied by intraosseous retrograde flow. For this reason, scaphoid waist fractures can interrupt the fragile blood flow to the proximal pole.

EPIDEMIOLOGY

The true incidence in Europe or elsewhere is difficult to ascertain, as not everyone with a scaphoid fracture will seek medical help. The reported incidence varies depending on the cases and the population. It has been reported in various countries in

The authors have nothing to disclose.
University Hospitals of Leicester, Gwendolen Road, Leicester LE5 4PW, UK
* Corresponding author.
E-mail address: jd96@leicester.ac.uk

Hand Clin 33 (2017) 501–509
http://dx.doi.org/10.1016/j.hcl.2017.04.003

Europe. In Denmark, the annual incidence is 22 in 100,000.[2] In Norway, the annual incidence is 43 in 100,000.[3] In Scotland, the annual reported incidence is 29 in 100,000,[4] and in the United Kingdom the incidence is 12.4 in 100,000.[5] This variability in incidence may reflect confounding factors, such as differences in age groups, climate, socioeconomic status, populations, and sporting interests. The lowest incidence among European countries is reported in the United Kingdom. There are a variety of possible explanations for this; for example, the definition of cases and population is clear, in Norway, the weather is colder, pavements icier, and more people ski and skate.[5] In contrast, the US military has an annual incidence of 121 scaphoid fractures in 100,000. This significantly higher incidence can be due to a younger, largely male population in the military, having easier access to urgent heath care facilities.

Hove[3] described scaphoid fractures occurring at a mean age of 25 years; 82% of fractures occurred in male individuals. Male individuals aged 15 to 29 years are at higher risk of sustaining scaphoid fractures. Girls aged 10 to 14 years have the highest incidence of scaphoid fractures among female individuals, as they are more likely to be involved in sporting activities. Schernberg[7] described these fractures as commonly occurring in the young, most active members of society, and that this population did not have the patience for immobilization in a cast. In the United Kingdom, those with a lower socioeconomic status are more likely to sustain hand trauma.[8] These injuries peak in the summer and autumn. Scaphoid waist fractures are the most frequent type of fracture. In the United Kingdom approximately 70% of these fractures occur at the waist, 20% at the distal pole, and 5% at the proximal pole. Although there is a lot of discrepancy in the literature as to where the proximal pole of the scaphoid begins, we have defined this as the proximal 20% of the scaphoid.[9,10]

MECHANISM OF INJURY

The most common mechanism of injury is forceful wrist hyperextension, usually from a fall onto an outstretched wrist. Middle-third scaphoid fractures are probably caused by extreme wrist extension with compression of the radial side of the palm.[11] Falls backward with the hand directed anteriorly are more likely to cause extreme wrist extension.[12] Less commonly a direct blow to the wrist also can cause a fracture.

CLASSIFICATION

Classification systems are based on the orientation and location of the fractures. The Russe classification uses the inclination of the fracture line to predict instability.[13] These are subclassified into horizontal oblique, transverse, or vertical oblique. Vertical oblique fractures are considered unstable, owing to greater shear forces across the fracture site, whereas horizontal oblique and transverse fractures have greater compressive force and are less likely to displace.

The Herbert classification[14] defines fractures as being stable or unstable and includes delayed union and nonunion (**Table 1**). This classification identifies types A to D. Type A fractures are stable acute fractures, and type B are unstable acute fractures. Although type A fractures typically can be treated nonoperatively, the other types of fracture usually require treatment.

The Mayo classification[15] also produces criteria for instability, it considers fractures with more than

Table 1
Herbert classification of scaphoid fractures

Site of Fracture	Type of Fracture	Description
Tuberosity	Type A (Stable)	A1: Tubercle A2: Incomplete
Waist fracture	Type B (Unstable)	B1: Oblique distal third B2: Displaced B4: Fracture dislocations
	Type C	Delayed union 6 wk after plaster
	Type D	D1: Fibrous nonunion D2: Sclerotic nonunion D3: Nonunion with fixed dorsal intercalated segmental instability
Proximal pole fracture	Type B3	Proximal third
	Type D4	Nonunion with avascular necrosis

Adapted from Singh HP, Dias JJ. Scaphoid fractures. J Bone Joint Surg Br 2011: 2; with permission.

1 mm of displacement, a lateral intrascaphoid angle greater than 350, bone loss or comminution, a perilunate fracture dislocation, dorsal intercalated segmental instability, malalignment, and fracture of the proximal pole as unstable. Associated soft tissue injuries are not considered in these classifications but clinicians are aware of these.

In Europe, the definition of displacement is largely similar to that in the rest of the world. The 4 bony features of displacement are shift, gap, angulation, and rotation. A fracture is considered displaced if the shift is greater than or equal to 1 mm, usually at the radial or dorsal cortical surface, on any radiographic view. A gap of more than 1 mm between the fragments seen on any radiograph or on sagittal or coronal computed tomography (CT) planes indicates instability and increase the risk of nonunion. Radiographs can be used to identify a gap, a step or tilting of the lunate, but with only moderate interobserver reliability.[16,17]

Angulation, typically into flexion, at the fracture site can be measured by using the dorsal cortical angle, lateral intrascaphoid angle, and height-to-length ratio.[18] The dorsal cortical angle is defined as the angle between tangential lines drawn along the flattest portion of the dorsal cortices of the proximal and distal scaphoid fragments on a lateral view. An angle greater than 1600 is considered abnormal. A mean dorsal cortical angle of 1390 as calculated on CT scans is considered normal.[19] The lateral intrascaphoid angle (LISA) is the angle between lines drawn perpendicular to the proximal and distal articular surfaces of scaphoid on posteroanterior (PA) or sagittal views. A study by Amadio and colleagues,[20] who used CT to study this angle, suggested 350 as a cutoff value. Patients in this study who had a higher LISA angle had a poor functional outcome. Due to overlap from other carpal bones, it is very difficult to quantify the intrascaphoid angulation. The mean height-to-length ratios calculated on longitudinal CT scaphoid sagittal scans of normal scaphoids is 0.60[16,20]; values greater than 0.65 are considered abnormal.

CLINICAL DIAGNOSIS

The diagnosis of a scaphoid fracture is usually suggested by the mechanism of injury, patient's age, and initial signs and symptoms. Swelling over the anatomic snuffbox increases the chances of a scaphoid fracture. Clinical signs include tenderness overlying the anatomic snuffbox or tenderness over the scaphoid tubercle and pain on applying axial pressure on the first metacarpal bone. These 3 together are reported to be 100% sensitive, but lack specificity (**Table 2**).

Table 2
Accuracy of clinical tests in diagnosis of scaphoid fractures

Clinical Tests	Specificity, %	Sensitivity, %
Snuffbox tenderness	40	90
Effusion (on ultrasound)	91	50
Tenderness over scaphoid tubercle	57	87
Scaphoid compression test	92	94
Combined	74	100

From Singh HP, Dias JJ. Scaphoid fractures. J Bone Joint Surg Br 2011: 1; with permission.

IMAGING

There are several different imaging modalities that can detect a scaphoid fracture. Several different radiographic views have been suggested for the scaphoid. Russe[13] originally suggested 4 views in 1960. These include PA, lateral, and 2 oblique views taken in 450 of supination and pronation respectively. In 1973, Ziter[21] proposed an ulna deviation view, which gives an elongated projection of the scaphoid; it is common to include this or a variant. Of the 4 Russe views, the most useful in diagnosing a scaphoid fracture are the PA and pronation oblique. Initial radiographs detect a fracture in up to 85% to 90%.[22] After 10 to 14 days, even on repeated good-quality radiographs, a scaphoid fracture can be missed, as the additional sensitivity is low. If CT is readily available, it can be used to rule out a scaphoid fracture. However, this does depend on the presence of trabecular or cortical disruption at the site of injury. The sensitivity of a CT is lower compared with bone scintigraphy. MRI can be used in the diagnosis and has been gaining popularity with the sensitivity being reported as 100%. It is more specific than a bone scan and has a higher interobserver agreement in case of fracture. Ultrasound is not usually done, although high-resolution ultrasounds can identify cortical disruption, radiocarpal effusion, and scaphoid-trapezium-trapezoid effusion, indicating a fracture. It is user dependent.

TREATMENT
Conservative Management: Plaster Casting Techniques

In an occult or a stable fracture, cast immobilization is the treatment of choice. Immobilization in a plaster cast for 4 to 6 weeks will lead to healing in 90% to 95% of scaphoid waist fractures; those that are displaced have a higher nonunion rate and may unite with a humpback deformity.

Clay and colleagues[23] in 1991 have shown that short arm casts with the thumb left free allows adequate immobilization of scaphoid fractures but permits the use of the hand and the elbow is not immobilized. Scaphoid union is not affected by the position of the wrist. A review article by Doornberg and colleagues[24] in 2011 showed no significant difference in above-elbow, below-elbow, scaphoid-type plaster cast (including the thumb), or Colles-type plaster cast (not including the thumb). The thumb need not be immobilized in scaphoid waist fractures. In Sweden, 90% of minimally or nondisplaced waist fractures were treated adequately with 6 weeks of plaster cast immobilization. Fractures with displacement of greater than 1.5 mm can heal within 6 to 10 weeks of conservative treatment.

The duration of immobilization can vary and depends on the type of fracture and assessment on repeated radiological examination, which allows an estimation of fracture union. In most undisplaced and stable fractures, 4 to 6 weeks of immobilization is sufficient. This method of treatment is reliable and successful, with low costs and a low complication rate. However, the disadvantages of cast immobilization are patient inconvenience and work restrictions.

Suspected Scaphoid Fractures

There is no standard approach to the management of suspected scaphoid fractures. A scaphoid fracture is suspected in a patient who has had a significant extension injury of the wrist, and has pain and tenderness on the radial aspect of the wrist but whose adequate radiographs do not show a scaphoid fracture.

Management of these patients includes placing them in either a removable splint or a below-elbow plaster cast. It is important to inform these patients of the possibility of a fracture and nonunion (10%). After 2 to 3 weeks, patients may be reviewed to see whether they still have clinical features suggestive of a scaphoid fracture. If swelling, tenderness in the anatomic snuffbox, or reduced grip is present, further radiographs or other imaging is obtained. In practice, radiographs are obtained first; if these are not clearly suggestive of a fracture, then a CT scan of the scaphoid with multiplanar reconstruction can often rule out a scaphoid fracture. Some units in Europe are exploring the routine use of CT or MRI in the early decision-making process for these patients.

Minimally Displaced Fractures

When deciding on the treatment of these fractures, it is important to take patient factors into consideration and to carefully discuss both the benefits and risks of conservative and surgical management. Schernberg[7] suggests percutaneous stabilization for those patients for whom early return to work or sport is a primary concern. Clementson and colleagues[25] have similar recommendations in the treatment of nondisplaced or minimally displaced scaphoid waist fractures, and in those patients for whom a quick return to work or sport is important, they offer arthroscopically assisted screw fixation. When treating acute undisplaced and minimally displaced waist fractures, the best evidence suggests that when comparing percutaneous fixation with plaster cast treatment there is faster union and earlier return to work and sport by approximately 7 weeks with similar union rates.[26,27] However, Dias and colleagues[28] conclude that on comparing open reduction and internal fixation (ORIF) with plaster casting, that there is no difference in the time taken to return to work with function being similar in the long term. There is a difference, however, when looking at people in different occupations. After ORIF, manual workers are able to return to work much earlier than after cast treatment; this results in a reduction in work disability costs. For nonmanual workers, plaster cast treatment has advantages over ORIF, as almost 40% of them are able to return to work with a cast.

Schädel-Höpfner and colleagues[29] advise that only stable and nondisplaced scaphoid fractures can be treated conservatively, and all other fractures need internal fixation with restoration of bone alignment. Rates of bone union for both nonoperative management and surgery are greater than 90%. Systematic reviews have shown that there are no differences in union rate or time to return to work and that any surgical benefits are short lived.[25,26] Plaster casting is less costly compared with ORIF. However, surgery reduces immobilization time and patients may return to work sooner; this is also reflected in a review article in 2010 by Buijze and colleagues.[30] Even though the risk of nonunion is higher with casting, there is up to a 30% complication rate with ORIF, including a long-term risk of arthritis.[31] There is, therefore, much variation in decision-making approaches for acute scaphoid fractures in Europe.

Displaced Fractures

These fractures have a higher risk of nonunion. They can be treated conservatively in a plaster cast but can malunite. Whether this is clinically significant in most cases is unclear. These fractures benefit from reduction of the fracture fragments and then stable internal fixation. Waist fractures that have more than 1 mm displacement in any direction are considered unstable and may require better stabilization than that provided by a plaster cast, as they have a nonunion rate 4 times that of undisplaced fractures. For displaced waist fractures, there is a reported 17 times greater likelihood of a nonunion when treated in a plaster cast compared with operative management.[18]

The palmar approach to the scaphoid limits injury to the blood supply of the scaphoid. Most proximal fractures are easily accessed through a dorsal exposure. Headless screws have gained popularity in the fixation of scaphoid fractures, and are almost universally used in Europe. Cannulated screw fixation can be used for both open and percutaneous fixation. Kirschner wires can be inserted into each fracture fragment to reduce the fracture. Central screw placement shortens time to union, but this may often not be possible because of the anatomy of the fracture and the bone.

Proximal Pole Fractures

Proximal pole fractures behave differently (**Fig. 1**). Five percent of scaphoid fractures are in the proximal fifth of the scaphoid. They are relatively uncommon injuries with few reports of their outcomes. These fractures have the poorest prognosis. The proximal pole has a precarious blood supply. This results in the high incidence of osteonecrosis and nonunion after proximal pole fractures (**Fig. 2**). Prolonged healing times of up to 6 months have been associated with cast treatment and a nonunion rate of up to 34% noted.[9] The rates of healing following nonunion surgery for proximal pole fractures[32] are particularly poor; this emphasizes importance

to achieving union in acute fractures. All these factors favor treating proximal pole fractures operatively. The union rate after ORIF is 66%.[9] The particular concerns with these fractures relate to the small size and relative avascularity of the proximal fragment. Arsalan-Werner and colleagues[33] recommend that proximal pole fractures should be treated operatively with screw fixation from the dorsal approach to avoid injury to the palmar carpal ligament and the blood supply to the scaphoid. Krimmer[34] also believes that all acute proximal pole fractures should be treated with ORIF.

The size of the proximal pole determines the type of fixation. A large fragment can be fixed with a headless compression screw. The starting point and placement of the screw is important (**Fig. 3**). The starting point should be proximal and dorsal to obtain central purchase on the proximal fragment. If the fragment is small, then Kirschner wires can be used to hold the fracture reduced, and if needed, transarticular fixation may be required (**Fig. 4**).

TECHNIQUES AND COMPLICATIONS OF SURGICAL FIXATION
Open Reduction and Internal Fixation

This method is used if the reduction of the fracture with closed methods is not possible. A variety of fixation methods are used in Europe, usually using some form of headless compression screw or cannulated systems.[35] The implant must be advanced below the cartilage at both ends of the scaphoid to prevent cartilage attrition of the radio-scaphoid or scaphoid-trapezium joints. The screw length is normally approximately 4 mm shorter than the measured length. A review article by Arsalan-Werner and colleagues[33] in Berlin suggests the use of a locking plate when screw osteosynthesis is not possible; for example, in wedge and multifragmentary fractures. The evidence for this is scanty.[36]

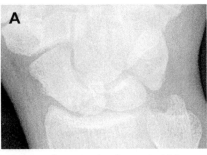 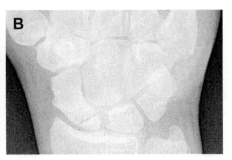

Fig. 1. Radiographs of proximal pole scaphoid fracture seen on 2 views. Note the horizontal orientation of this fracture with the ulnar end of the fracture extending into the scapholunate joint. (A) 45 degree semi prone view and (B) posterior-anterior view of the scaphoid demonstrating a proximal pole fracture.

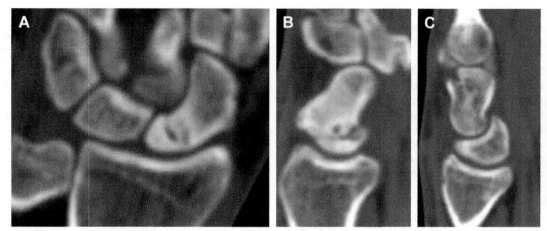

Fig. 2. CT scan of a scaphoid proximal pole nonunion. Multiplanar reconstructions in the sagittal (*B*) and coronal (*A*) planes of the scaphoid and a sagittal plane of the wrist (*C*) showing a proximal pole fracture nonunion with tilting of the lunate into a dorsal intercalated segment instability pattern. The latter may be due to scapholunate instability as the proximal scaphoid is not tilted.

Complications During or Relating to Surgery

Mostly, complications are related to the wound (15%), including sensitivity, hypertrophic scar, wound infection (<1%), and cutaneous nerve dysesthesia. These may be less with the percutaneous technique. Nonunion is an important risk (5%–7%); it is imperative that this risk should be discussed during the consenting process. Complex regional pain syndrome is uncommon, occurring in approximately 3%.[28] This can also happen after nonoperative treatment. Other complications include injury to the palmar cutaneous branch of the median nerve (2%).[31] Failure of surgical technique, for example, breakage of metalwork, implant protrusion into adjacent joints, and intraoperative injury to joints, nerves, or tendons can compromise outcomes.

Postoperative Care and Rehabilitation

This is adjusted for the individual patient and pattern of fracture. Generally, a bulky bandage or a Futuro splint is used to protect the hand following surgery. A below-elbow plaster cast may be used for approximately 6 weeks followed

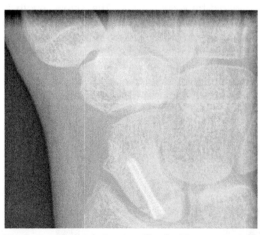

Fig. 3. Proximal pole fracture fixed with an antegrade headless screw. The screw position is eccentric with a tenuous hold of the proximal fragment. The entry point could be improved by siting it at the junction of the lunate surface and the radius surface of the scaphoid. The fracture line is still identifiable. This fracture subsequently united, although quite slowly.

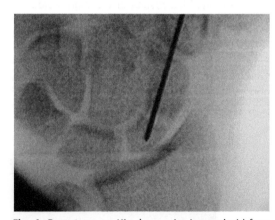

Fig. 4. Percutaneous Kirschner wire in scaphoid fracture. This can be introduced in a retrograde manner into the distal fragment, can assist correction of a minor step, and then advanced into the proximal fragment. Once good reduction is confirmed on image intensifier, a cannulated headless screw of appropriate length can be introduced to secure reduction and compress the fracture.

by a Futuro splint. Prolonged cast immobilization beyond 8 weeks is usually not needed. For athletes,[37] modification of treatment programs has been carried out; for example, fiberglass casts are exchanged for soft or padded casts on game days. These are to minimize the potential injury to other athletes. Providing treatment is not delayed, the modification of treatment programs for athletes has not caused a problem with union.[33] In general, however, patients are advised against contact sports for 2 to 3 months, and they are informed of the risks of refracture.

OUTCOMES
Healing Rates and Symptoms

Before 12 weeks, union rates based on radiographic evaluation are unreliable. Studies that have assessed union at 6 months or a year are much more reliable. Although a good outcome is presumed after union; injury to articular cartilage and alteration to the carpal dynamics can result in persistent pain and secondary osteoarthritis. The European experience is that tenderness and pain are reported after a united fracture in up to 20% of patients at 1.7 to 2.8 years, but both wrist movement and grip strength are nearly normal.[17] Secondary osteoarthritis is seen in 5%, 7 years after fracture union. For fractures of the waist following cast treatment, union rates approach 90%. In proximal pole fractures, nonunion occurs in a third; it is rare in distal fractures.

Complications

Malunion
This is usually a flexion deformity of the scaphoid but can also be an ulnar translation or pronation of the distal fragment.[38] This can be seen either as a flexion or humpback deformity; special imaging may be required to detect this. The effect of this on wrist function is unclear. Cadaver studies that simulated scaphoid malunion show reduced wrist extension proportional to the angular deformity. However, clinical studies have demonstrated that mild malunion is well tolerated. Nonunion that is treated can lead to malunion with a humpback deformity, which may impair function and restrict movement; it is unclear whether it leads to early osteoarthritis. The role of corrective osteotomy is controversial and only done in a few units in Europe.

Nonunion
Nonunion is defined as a fracture, given sufficient time has not united and will not unite without intervention. Following conservative treatment, the incidence of nonunion in scaphoid fractures is 12.3%. Prosser and Isbister[39] identified 4 different patterns of presentation:

1. Patients treated and followed up adequately in whom radiographs reveal nonunion
2. Patients treated but followed up inadequately; that is, the patient is discharged prematurely thinking the fracture has united, however he or she re-presents with a nonunion
3. Patients who were never treated because they did not consult a doctor, they present later with a symptomatic nonunion, often after a further injury
4. Patients in whom nonunion is an incidental finding when examination is undertaken for a different reason

Not all nonunions are symptomatic, 30% of patients at the time of diagnosis are free of symptoms. Untreated, symptoms eventually develop in almost all patients, although this can be several years after injury. Patients may have radial and dorsal swelling and tenderness. The scaphoid tuberosity can also be tender to palpation, with pain felt at the extremes of extension. It is common for these patients to have loss of wrist extension due to carpal collapse and palmar capsular contracture.[40]

The diagnosis is usually confirmed on radiographs. A clear gap at the fracture site denotes nonunion.[41] Commonly, a fracture line may still be visible with some partial consolidation ("partially united"); in these cases a CT scan can help confirm the degree of union.[42] Generally, scaphoid nonunion affects the young and active patient. Left untreated, pain and osteoarthritis are usual consequences. Surgery is therefore indicated in both symptomatic and asymptomatic cases. A careful assessment of the degree of osteoarthritis should be made; if significant arthritis is present, consideration of salvage surgery may be more appropriate. The aims of surgery are to achieve union, reduce the incidence of osteoarthritis, improve function, and eradicate symptoms. Surgery usually involves bone grafting with or without internal fixation. Assessment of the nonunion is made on radiographic and CT examination and intraoperative examination. Bone grafts can be either vascularized or nonvascularized. Nonvascularized bone grafting with or without fixation has reported union rates of 70% to 80%. Vascularized bone grafting restores blood supply, promotes primary bone healing, and maintains structural integrity. Mathoulin and Haerle[43] advocate the use of vascularized bone graft in nonunion and have seen rapid union. Mostly, for scaphoid waist nonunions without adverse features, such as avascular necrosis, failed previous surgery, long duration of nonunion, or proximal pole nonunion, a nonvascularized bone graft is probably sufficient and commonly done in Europe. If bone grafting fails, then future surgery is likely to be unsuccessful. Worse results are seen with proximal fractures, increasing duration of nonunion and avascular necrosis of the proximal pole.

SUMMARY

The European approach to the treatment of scaphoid fractures is for most to be treated in a plaster cast for approximately 6 weeks. Acute/primary surgery may be considered in patients with displaced scaphoid fractures, proximal pole fractures, fractures associated with perilunate deformity, open fractures, and patients with multiple injuries. However, decision making is not uniform across Europe. The European literature stresses the importance of taking the patient's wishes into consideration after careful counseling about alternative treatment methods.

REFERENCES

1. Rhemrev SJ, Ootes D, Beeres FJ, et al. Current methods of diagnosis and treatment of scaphoid fractures. Int J Emerg Med 2011;4:4.
2. Larsen CM, Brondum V, Skov O. Epidemiology of scaphoid fractures in Odense, Denmark. Acta Orthop Scand 1992;63:216–8.
3. Hove LM. Epidemiology of scaphoid fractures in Bergen, Norway. Scand J Plast Reconstr Surg Hand Surg 1999;33:423–6.
4. Duckworth AD, Jenkins PJ, Aitken SA, et al. Scaphoid fracture epidemiology. J Trauma Acute Care Surg 2012;72:e41–5.
5. Garala K, Taub NA, Dias JJ. The epidemiology of fractures of the scaphoid: impact of age, gender, deprivation and seasonality. Bone Joint J 2016;98:654–9.
6. Available at: http://www.boneandjoint.org.uk/content/focus/scaphoid-fractures.
7. Schernberg F. Fractures recentes du scaphoide (moins de trois semaines). Chir Main 2005;24:117–31.
8. Horton TC, Dias JJ, Burke FD. Social deprivation and hand injury. J Hand Surg Br Vol 2007;32:256–61.
9. Eastley N, Singh H, Dias JJ, et al. Union rates after proximal scaphoid fractures; meta-analyses and review of available evidence. J Hand Surg Eur Vol 2013;38:888–97.
10. Ramamurthy C, Cutler L, Nuttall D, et al. The factors affecting outcome after non-vascular bone grafting and internal fixation for nonunion of the scaphoid. J Bone Joint Surg Br 2007;89:627–32.
11. Weber ER, Chao EY. An experimental approach to the mechanism of scaphoid waist fractures. J Hand Surg Am 1978;3:142–8.
12. Cockshott WP. Distal avulsion fractures of the scaphoid. Br J Radiol 1980;53:1037–40.
13. Russe O. Fracture of the carpal navicular. Diagnosis, nonoperative treatment and operative treatment. J Bone Joint Surg Am 1960;42:759–68.
14. Herbert TJ, Fisher WE. Management of the fractured scaphoid using a new bone screw. J Bone Joint Surg Br 1984;66:114–23.
15. Cooney WP, Dobyns JH, Linscheid RL. Fractures of the scaphoid: a rational approach to management. Clin Orthop Relat Res 1980;149:90–7.
16. Bhat M, McCarthy M, Davis T, et al. MRI and plain radiography in the assessment of displaced fractures of the waist of the carpal scaphoid. Bone Joint J 2004;86:705–13.
17. Dias JJ, Brenkel IJ, Finlay DB. Patterns of union in fractures of the waist of the scaphoid. J Bone Joint Surg Br 1989;71:307–10.
18. Singh HP, Taub N, Dias JJ. Management of displaced fractures of the waist of the scaphoid: meta-analyses of comparative studies. Injury 2012;43:933–9.
19. Bain GI, Bennett JD, MacDermid JC, et al. Measurement of the scaphoid humpback deformity using longitudinal computed tomography: intra- and interobserver variability using various measurement techniques. J Hand Surg Am 1998;23:76–81.
20. Amadio PC, Berquist TH, Smith DK, et al. Scaphoid malunion. J Hand Surg Am 1989;14:679–87.
21. Ziter FM Jr. A modified view of the carpal navicular. Radiology 1973;108:706–7.
22. Hunter JC, Escobedo EM, Wilson AJ, et al. MR imaging of clinically suspected scaphoid fractures. Am J Roentgenol 1997;168:1287–93.
23. Clay NR, Dias JJ, Costigan PS, et al. Need the thumb be immobilised in scaphoid fractures? A randomised prospective trial. J Bone Joint Surg Br 1991;73:828–32.
24. Doornberg JN, Buijze GA, Ham SJ, et al. Nonoperative treatment for acute scaphoid fractures: a systematic review and meta-analysis of randomized controlled trials. J Trauma 2011;71:1073–81.
25. Clementson M, Jorgsholm P, Besjakov J, et al. Conservative treatment versus arthroscopic-assisted screw fixation of scaphoid waist fractures–a randomized trial with minimum 4-year follow-up. J Hand Surg Am 2015;40:1341–8.
26. Bond CD, Shin AY, McBride MT, et al. Percutaneous screw fixation or cast immobilization for nondisplaced scaphoid fractures. J Bone Joint Surg Am 2001;83:483–8.
27. McQueen MM, Gelbke MK, Wakefield A, et al. Percutaneous screw fixation versus conservative treatment for fractures of the waist of the scaphoid: a

prospective randomised study. J Bone Joint Surg Br 2008;90:66–71.

28. Dias JJ, Wildin CJ, Bhowal B, et al. Should acute scaphoid fractures be fixed? A randomized controlled trial. J Bone Joint Surg Am 2005;87:2160–8.

29. Schädel-Höpfner M, Prommersberger KJ, Eisenschenk A, et al. Treatment of carpal fractures. Recommendations of the hand surgery Group of the German Trauma Society. Der Unfallchirurg 2010;113:741–54 [in German].

30. Buijze GA, Doornberg JN, Ham JS, et al. Surgical compared with conservative treatment for acute nondisplaced or minimally displaced scaphoid fractures: a systematic review and meta-analysis of randomized controlled trials. J Bone Joint Surg Am 2010;92:1534–44.

31. Modi CS, Nancoo T, Powers D, et al. Operative versus nonoperative treatment of acute undisplaced and minimally displaced scaphoid waist fractures–a systematic review. Injury 2009;40:268–73.

32. Brogan DM, Moran SL, Shin AY. Outcomes of open reduction and internal fixation of acute proximal pole scaphoid fractures. Hand (N Y) 2015;10:227–32.

33. Arsalan-Werner A, Sauerbier M, Mehling IM. Current concepts for the treatment of acute scaphoid fractures. Eur J Trauma Emerg Surg 2016;42:3–10.

34. Krimmer H. Management of acute fractures and nonunions of the proximal pole of the scaphoid. J Hand Surg Br 2002;27:245–8.

35. Brauer RB, Dierking M, Werber KD. The use of the Herbert bone screw by the freehand-method for osteosynthesis scaphoid fracture. Der Unfallchirurg 1997;100:776–81.

36. Dias J, Brealey S, Choudhary S, et al. Scaphoid waist internal fixation for fractures trial (SWIFFT) protocol: a pragmatic multi-centre randomised controlled trial of cast treatment versus surgical fixation for the treatment of bi-cortical, minimally displaced fractures of the scaphoid waist in adults. BMC Musculoskelet Disord 2016;17:248.

37. Riester JN, Baker BE, Mosher JF, et al. A review of scaphoid fracture healing in competitive athletes. Am J Sports Med 1985;13:159–61.

38. Fernandez DL, Martin CJ, Gonzalez JP. Scaphoid malunion. The significance of rotational malalignment. J Hand Surg Br 1998;23:771–5.

39. Prosser GH, Isbister ES. The presentation of scaphoid non-union. Injury 2003;34:65–7.

40. Barton NJ. Twenty questions about scaphoid fractures. J Hand Surg Br 1992;17:289–310.

41. Dias JJ. Definition of union after acute fracture and surgery for fracture nonunion of the scaphoid. J Hand Surg Br 2001;26:321–5.

42. Clementson M, Jorgsholm P, Besjakov J, et al. Union of scaphoid waist fractures assessed by CT scan. J Wrist Surg 2015;4:49–55.

43. Mathoulin C, Haerle M. Vascularized bone graft from the palmar carpal artery for treatment of scaphoid nonunion. J Hand Surg Br 1998;23:318–23.

Carpal Ligaments
A Functional Classification

Marc Garcia-Elias, MD, PhD[a,b,*], Inma Puig de la Bellacasa, MD[b,c], Corinne Schouten, MD[d]

KEYWORDS

- Anatomy • Axial loading • Carpal ligaments • Kinetics • Wrist

KEY POINTS

- Carpal ligaments are not static cable-like collections of fibers holding bones together but complex bone-binding structures containing sensorial elements (mechanoreceptors) aimed at detecting changes in carpal bone position and transmitting that information to the sensorimotor system for a centralized control of wrist stability.
- Depending on the direction of its fascicles, some carpal ligaments are particularly set to detect intracarpal pronation torques. Grouped in the so-called helical antipronation ligaments they would be predominately active when the carpus is axially loaded, from distal to proximal, along the longitudinal axis of the hand, or when the distal row is torqued into pronation.
- The so-called helical antisupination ligaments (HASLs) are formed by ligaments that are especially active when the wrist is pulled distally or when the distal row is subjected to a supination torque. They may be subclassified into medial and lateral HASLs.

Until the late 1960s all painful wrists with radiographs that showed no bony injury were treated as sprains.[1,2] Textbooks did not pay much attention to isolated carpal ligament ruptures, and the occasional cases in which an apparently benign injury had progressed toward global joint deterioration and carpal collapse were considered exceptions, proving the rule that most sprained wrists healed uneventfully.[3] That changed dramatically in the early 1970s with the introduction of the concept of carpal instability by Geoffrey Fisk,[4] Linscheid and colleagues,[5] and Dobyns and colleagues.[6] Emphasizing the need for a thorough clinical and radiological examination, a variety of new conditions, formerly misdiagnosed as sprains,

were brought to light. This gave rise to an exponential increase of publications suggesting surgical techniques to reestablish function.[7–12] It did not take long for most surgeons to be convinced about the inevitability of an adverse evolution should these injuries be left untreated.[13,14] Preventive repair of all torn ligaments became common practice.[7,9,10] However, the problem was how to achieve a solid repair, when all that was left from a damaged interosseous ligament were 2 short, irregularly torn, often retracted ligament stumps. One option was to reinforce the repair with a capsulodesis,[7,15] another was to reconstruct those unrepairable ligaments with a free tendon graft, a tenodesis, or a bone-ligament-bone

Disclosure Statement: The authors do not have any relationship with a commercial company that has a direct financial interest in the subject matter or materials discussed in this article or with a company making a competing product.
[a] Hand & Upper Limb Surgery, Institut Kaplan, Passeig de la Bonanova, 9, 2on 2a, Barcelona 08022, Spain; [b] Department of Anatomy, Facultat de Medicina, Universitat de Barcelona, Carrer de Villarroel 170, Barcelona 08036, Spain; [c] Hand and Upper Extremity Surgery, Mútua de Terrassa Hospital Universitari, Plaça del Doctor Robert, 5, Terrassa 08221, Spain; [d] Department of Plastic and Reconstructive, Hand, and Aesthetic Surgery, Catharina Hospital Eindhoven, Vondelstraat 75H, Nijmegen 6512BD, The Netherlands
* Corresponding author. Institut Kaplan, Passeig de la Bonanova, 9, 2on 2a, Barcelona 08022, Spain.
E-mail address: garciaelias@institut-kaplan.com

hand.theclinics.com

transplant.[11,12,16–21] Attractive from a technical perspective, most hand surgeons sooner or later gave these reconstructions a try. The results used to be modest if not completely disappointing.[22,23] Indeed, the complexity of a ligament cannot be expected to be easily substituted by a piece of avascular tendon. It is not surprising that these injured wrists seldom if ever regained normal alignment and full function.

With time it was learned that not all ligament tears become painful and dysfunctional, and that the incidence of asymptomatic scapholunate ligament ruptures is not low.[24–26] Carpal instability is more than a ligament deficiency problem. It is a multifactorial phenomenon involving inadequate wrist proprioception, poor interaction between ligaments and muscles, and lack of control of the entire process by the sensorimotor system.[27–31]

This article updates the role of carpal ligaments in this process, including a new kinetic classification of carpal ligaments based on their behavior under different isometric loading conditions. The goal is to improve understanding of the mechanisms of carpal stabilization and to find reliable solutions when these mechanisms have failed.

This article does not cover all aspects of ligament function. It is only a review of the stabilizing role of ligaments from a kinetic perspective. The role of ligaments ensuring adequate carpal kinematics is a different subject also worth revisiting. The ligaments of the carpometacarpal joints are not discussed.

INTERNAL STRUCTURE OF CARPAL LIGAMENTS

Most carpal ligaments have a core of densely packed collagen fibers (fascicular region), surrounded by a layer of well-vascularized, loose connective tissue (epifascicular region).[32–35] Within the epifascicular region, and close to its insertion sites, variable amounts of Ruffini, Pacinian or Golgi corpuscles are found.[28,36] These so-called mechanoreceptors are surrounded by a network of dendritic projections emerging from the nearby nerves. The densely packed fibers of the fascicular region are meant to keep joint motion within its normal limits (primary stabilization). When the limits of normal joint movement are breached, the sensory corpuscles generate afferent stimuli, which are transferred to the central nervous system. Once in the dorsal horn of the spinal cord, the stimuli continue up the dorsolateral and spinocerebellar tracts for final analysis by the cerebellum, or return to the wrist in the form of a monosynaptic reflex. This will activate an adequate response by the muscles, especially the ultimate wrist stabilizers.[27,28]

Most ligaments play both mechanical and sensory roles in maintaining carpal stability. However, not all ligaments are equally active in both roles. Some ligaments mainly have a static constraining function, whereas others have a predominantly proprioceptive function.[35] The first are characterized by the presence of tightly packed collagen fibers and a limited number of sensory corpuscles. The second have a less compact arrangement of collagen fibers but a reasonably dense population of mechanoreceptors. Although the mechanically important ligaments are primarily located in the lateral (scaphoid) load-bearing column, the important sensory ligaments mainly insert onto the triquetrum. Based on this, the triquetrum has been considered the source of most of the proprioceptive information required to stabilize the joint. This should be kept in mind when planning excision of the triquetrum.[35]

ANATOMIC CLASSIFICATIONS OF CARPAL LIGAMENTS

The wrist is probably the joint with the largest variation in ligament sizes, fascicle orientations, and elastic properties in the human body.[32,37] From a morphologic point of view, carpal ligaments have been classified based on different parameters.

Classification by Location

Based on the location of the ligament relative to the joint capsule, a ligament may be extracapsular (located outside the wrist capsule), intracapsular (within the depth of the wrist capsule), or intra-articular (inside the joint cavity, usually covered by a thin layer of synovial tissue).[26,32] There are only 3 extracapsular ligaments: the transverse carpal ligament that forms the roof of the carpal tunnel and the 2 distal ligament connections of the pisiform, 1 to the hook of the hamate and the other to the base of the fifth metacarpal. The dorsal scapholunate interosseous ligament is an example of intra-articular ligament and the long radiolunate of an intracapsular ligament.

Classification by Joints

Depending on which articulations are being linked, ligaments have been classified into extrinsic, intrinsic, and interosseous.[26,32] Extrinsic ligaments connect the distal epiphyses of the radius and ulna with the carpal bones. Intrinsic ligaments bind carpal bones between different rows and interosseous ligaments connect adjacent bones within the same row. Aside from their topographic differences, the ligaments from these 3 categories differ in their elastic properties and modes of failure.

Extrinsic ligaments are long, quite elastic, and poorly resistant to high tension. Because of these features and because they insert mainly onto bone, they are more likely to suffer midsubstance ruptures than avulsions. Intrinsic ligaments, by contrast, are short ligaments that mainly insert onto cartilage and, therefore, suffer more avulsions than ruptures. The same applies to the interosseous ligaments, except that they are the shortest and stiffest of all.

Classification by Orientation

Ligaments of the wrist may be transverse, longitudinal, or oblique relative to the longitudinal axis of the hand.[26,32,37]

Transverse interosseous ligaments
Anatomic variations aside, the human wrist has 25 ligaments. Of those, 14 have an overall transverse orientation relative to the main axis of the forearm: 2 scaphotriquetral ligaments (palmar and dorsal), 10 interosseous ligaments (5 palmar and 5 dorsal: scapholunate, lunotriquetral, trapeziotrapezoid, trapezoid-capitate, and capitohamate), and 2 intra-articular ligaments within the trapezoid-capitate and capitohamate articulations. Their function is essentially dictated by the need of the rows to maintain a close kinematic relationship during motion.

Longitudinal ligaments
Only 3 ligaments have a vertical (longitudinal) orientation: the most radial (radioscaphoid) fascicle of the extrinsic radiocarpal ligaments (often referred to as the lateral or radial collateral ligament), the short radiolunate ligament, and the most ulnar (ulnotriquetral) fascicle of the extrinsic ulnocarpal ligaments (often referred to as the medial or ulnar collateral ligament). The stabilizing role of these ligaments is poorly understood.[32] When the wrist is loaded axially in a neutral position, none of these vertical ligaments become taut. Whether they would play a significant role when the wrist is isometrically loaded in extension is an interesting, yet untested conjecture. It is also possible that these ligaments represent a phylogenic vestige of the most important wrist stabilizers that allowed our ancestors to arm-swing from tree limb to tree limb. Further research is needed to clarify this.

Oblique ligaments
This is, by far, the most important group of ligaments in terms of wrist stability. It includes 8 ligaments with an oblique course relative to the main axis of the hand. The obliquity may be in 2 directions: from proximal-radial to distal-ulnar or from proximal-ulnar to distal-radial. On volar side, the first are set to resist intracarpal pronation torques, whereas the second become taut when the distal row is torqued in supination relative to the fixed radius. On the dorsal side, the opposite is correct. Based on this, it was proposed to call the first group antisupination ligaments and the second, antipronation ligaments.[31] The antisupination group of ligaments includes the dorsal radiotriquetral (radiocarpal) ligament, the volar ulnolunate ligament, the scaphotrapeziotrapezoid ligament, and the ulnar limb of the arcuate ligament (also known as the volar triquetrohamate-capitate ligament). The antipronation ligaments include the radioscaphocapitate ligament, the long radiolunate ligament, the dorsal intercarpal ligament, and the volar scaphocapitate ligament.

CARPAL LIGAMENT DYNAMICS (KINETICS)

Dynamics (also known as kinetics) is the branch of physics that deals with the effects of forces on the material bodies, in this case, the carpal ligaments.[38,39] In the laboratory, a wrist is said to be axially loaded when there is an external force applied from distal to proximal, along the long (middle) finger metacarpal, with the wrist in neutral.[31,39] The magnitude and direction of carpal displacements depends on the shape of the articular surfaces, and the status of the different soft tissue constraints (capsule, ligaments, and muscles).[38] When the wrist is loaded axially, ligaments may become taut, remain unchanged, or relax. When 2 ligaments exhibit a similar response, these ligaments are said to have an isodynamic behavior.

In theory, mechanoreceptors within isodynamic ligaments generate similar proprioceptive stimuli at about the same time. This is particularly helpful when a ligament is torn. The sensorimotor system does not know what happens within that ligament; yet, the information provided by its isodynamic partners is used as an equivalent of the stimuli that would be generated by the damaged ligament, should it be intact. This is the trick used to maintain stability in the area. Indeed, ligament integrity is not a requirement for the wrist to be stable, as long as their isodynamic partners provide the missing information.

To investigate ligament isodynamics, 8 fresh cadaver arms were tested in a specially designed jig that allowed measurement of carpal bone displacement under different loading conditions (**Fig. 1**).[29] The goal was to identify groups of ligaments with similar behavior (isodynamic ligaments) under 2 different loading conditions (axial load and axial traction).

To quantify changes in ligament tightness, a dedicated ligament tensiometer would have been

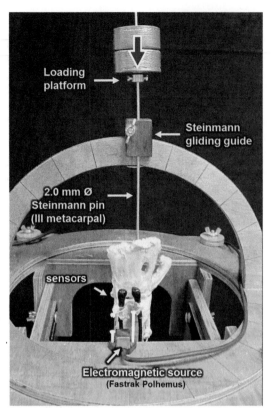

Fig. 1. The testing apparatus used to investigate ligament synergies in the axially loaded wrist. A 2 mm Ø Steinmann pin inserted in the third metacarpal, a loading platform, a pin-gliding guide, and an electromagnetic motion tracking device (FASTRAK [Polhemus, Colchester, Vermont, USA]) were used to measure attempted displacements induced by isometrically loading the wrist (*red arrow*) or by axially distracting the third metacarpal away from the radius. (*Courtesy of* Polhemus, Colchester, VT.)

ideal. Unfortunately, the ones available were not small enough to be used in the wrist and did not provide real-time tension determinations in the ranges expected in the carpus. Less ideal, but still more reliable than manually testing fiber tensions with a hook, is the so-called attempted carpal displacements method.[39] It is not a quantitative method but it helps identify ligament synergies in the wrist under different loading conditions.

From those studies, it was learned that when the wrist is axially loaded the carpal bones move with reasonably consistent patterns.[29–31,38] The distal carpal row always pronates, the scaphoid always flexes, and the lunate joint slides down the volar-ulnar slope of the distal radius (**Fig. 2**). The triquetrum may flex or extend with the latter tending to predominate (**Fig. 3**).

When the wrist is subjected to axial traction along the long finger metacarpal, the entire carpus

translocates distally and radially toward the dorsoradial rim of the radius, whereas the distal carpal row undergoes a supination rotation; the scaphoid extends; and the triquetrum, constrained palmarly by the ulnocarpal ligaments, rotates into flexion.

KINETIC CLASSIFICATION OF CARPAL LIGAMENTS

When axially loaded, the properly constrained carpal bones do not displace beyond normal limits.[38,39] Ligaments are responsible for that. Most ligaments cannot, however, control multidirectional instabilities. They can only constrain unidirectional displacements. Consequently, if the displacement is known, which ligaments must be in charge of that particular displacement can be estimated. **Table 1** contains the list of attempted displacements detected for the axially loaded wrist and the axially tractioned wrist, as well as the most likely combination of ligaments that constrain such displacements.

From those kinetic studies, the following was learned:

1. Transverse interosseous ligaments are only indirectly involved in the stabilization of the axially loaded wrist; their function is mainly directed to maintaining normal relationships between bones of the same row.
2. Vertical ligaments are not necessary to maintain carpal stability in neutral position; whether they are more active in other positions is not clear.
3. The most important stabilizing ligaments are arranged following 2 different helical patterns (**Fig. 4**).[31]

Based on this latter finding, the authors submit that, from a kinetic perspective, there are 2 major groups of carpal ligaments: helical antipronation and helical antisupination.

Helical Antipronation Ligaments

As previously stated, when the wrist is subjected to an axial compression, the distal row pronates, the scaphoid flexes, the triquetrum extends, and the entire carpus tends to slide down the ulnopalmar slope of the distal radius. The most effective ligaments to constrain all these attempted displacements are

1. The long radiolunate ligament that prevents ulnar translocation
2. The palmar and dorsal lunotriquetral ligaments that prevent triquetrum extension

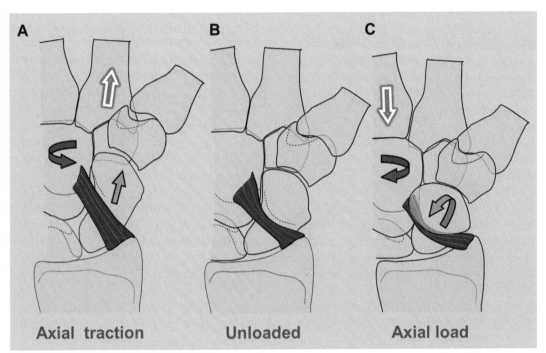

Fig. 2. Attempted displacements measured in the scaphoid column in 3 loading conditions. (*A*) Axial traction (*white arrow*) consistently provoked supination of the distal row (*orange arrow*) and extension and distal migration of the scaphoid (*blue straight arrow*). (*B*) Scaphoid motion is always mediated by the presence of the oblique radioscaphocapitate (RSC) ligament (*in red*). (*C*) When axially loaded (*white straight arrow*), the distal row always pronates (*curved orange arrow*) and the scaphoid rotates into flexion and pronation (*blue curved arrow*) around the oblique RSC ligament.

3. The dorsal scaphotriquetral and dorsal scapholunate ligaments that prevent flexion and pronation of the scaphoid
4. The radioscaphocapitate and scaphocapitate ligaments that prevent excessive distal row pronation (**Fig. 5**).

In other words, to avoid carpal collapse under axial compressive loads, the wrist needs 3 oblique and 4 transverse ligaments arranged as a helix around the capitate. It is the so-called helical antipronation ligaments (HAPLs), a group of isodynamic ligaments, that start on the volar side of the radial styloid process and winds around the central column of the wrist to insert distally on the volar aspect of the capitate. If the sensorimotor system works properly, the HAPLs act as the first line of defense against the carpal collapse induced by an axial compressive load or by its equivalent hyperpronation torque of the distal carpal row relative to a fixed forearm. Failure of the HAPLs would result in an instability affecting mostly the lateral column of the wrist, the most frequent being scapholunate instability.[29–31] From this viewpoint, the ideal treatment of the severe scapholunate instability associated with a

translocation of the lunate is that which reconstructs not only the primary stabilizers but also the entire HAPL group. This is the so-called spiral antipronation tenodeses. The first cases published by Chee and colleagues[21] (2012) are very promising.

Helical Antisupination Ligaments

When the carpus is stressed by a distally directed traction force, or by its equivalent, a hypersupination torque to the distal row, there is a group of isodynamic ligaments, similarly arranged as a helix, designed to constrain such destabilizing force.[31] They are called helical antisupination ligaments (HASLs) and can be differentiated into 2 groups: the medial and the lateral HASLs (**Fig. 6**):

• The medial HASLs embrace the ulnar corner of the wrist and include the dorsal radiotriquetral (radiocarpal) ligament and the palmar triquetrohamate-capitate ligament (ulnar limb of the arcuate ligament). A medial HASL failure would result in a palmar midcarpal instability.

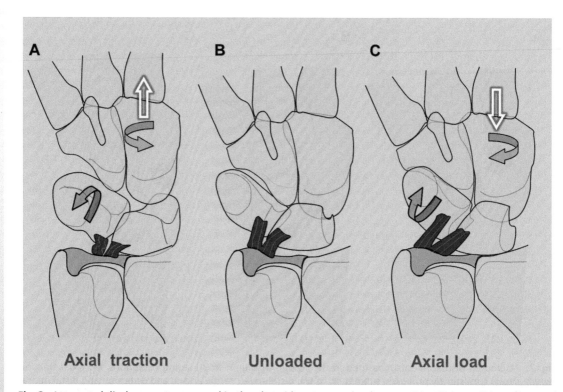

Fig. 3. Attempted displacements measured in the ulnarside carpus under the same 3 loading conditions discussed in **Fig. 2.** (*A*) Axial traction (*white arrow*) consistently provoked supination of the distal row (*green arrow*) and flexion of the triquetrum (*curved blue arrow*). (*B*) Lunate and triquetrum motion is mediated by the ulnocarpal ligaments (*in red*). (*C*) When axially loaded (*white straight arrow*) the distal row pronates (*curved green arrow*) and the triquetrum rotates into flexion and supination (*blue curved arrow*).

Table 1
Kinetic analysis of 8 human cadaver wrists under 2 isometric loading conditions (axial loading and axial traction)

	Axial Loading	Axial Traction
Distal row	*Pronation* SC[a] RSC[a]	*Supination* TqHC[b]
Scaphoid	*Flexion* Dorsal SL[a] Dorsal STq[a]	*Extension* STT[c] Volar SL[c]
Triquetrum	*Extension* Volar LTq[a] Dorsal LTq[a]	*Flexion* Dorsal RTq[b]
Lunate	*Ulnar translocation* Long RL[a]	*Radial translocation* UL[c]

Included are the most predominant attempted displacements registered (in italics), and the most likely ligament constrains for each bone and loading condition.

Abbreviations: LTq, lunotriquetral; RL, radiolunate; RSC, radioscaphocapitate; RTq, radiotriquetral; SC, scaphocapitate; SL, scapholunate; STq, scaphotriquetral; STT, scaphotrapeziotrapezoidal; TqHC, triquetrohamate-capitate; UL, ulnolunate.

[a] Helical antipronation ligament.
[b] Medial helical antisupination ligament.
[c] Lateral helical antisupination ligament.

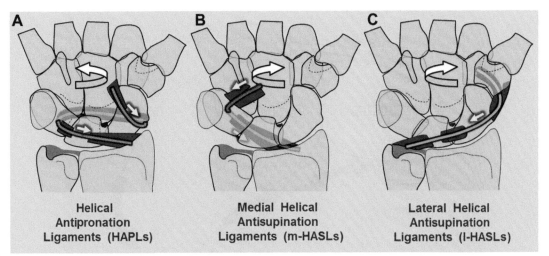

Fig. 4. Three groups of ligaments each play a specific role in the primary stabilization of the axially loaded carpus. (A) The helical antipronation ligaments become simultaneously taut (*yellow arrows*) when the distal row is torqued in pronation (*curved white arrow*). (B) The medial helical antisupination ligaments (HASLs) resist (*yellow arrows*) the tendency of the ulnarside bones to translocate palmarly (*curved white arrow*). (C) The lateral HASLs become particularly active (*yellow straight arrow*) when the distal row is forced into supination (*curved white arrow*).

- The lateral HASLs cover the radial corner of the wrist and include the ulnocarpal ligament, the volar scapholunate ligament, and the dorsolateral scaphotrapezotrapezoidal ligament. Failure of the lateral HASL would cause scaphotrapezotrapezoidal instability, ulnocarpal instability, or both.

By depicting both the HAPLs and HASLs in a single drawing, it quickly comes to mind that these ligaments resemble a Chinese finger trap, which is a cylindrical braid made out of helical set of wires.[26,30] By pulling it distally, the braid lengthens but simultaneously narrows it (**Fig. 7**). This is the Chinese finger trap principle; that is, the more the braid is pulled

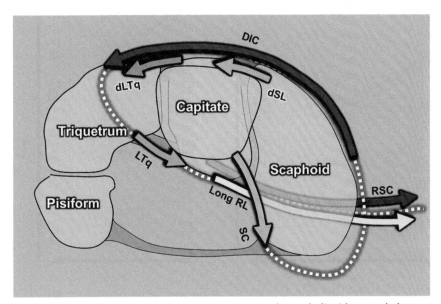

Fig. 5. Ligaments that constrain intracarpal pronation. Arranged as a helicoid around the central column, these ligaments (*multicolored arrows*) are the first line of defense against carpal collapse. DIC, dorsal intercarpal ligament; dLTq, dorsal lunotriquetral ligament; dSL, dorsal scapholunate ligament; Long RL, long radiolunate ligament; LTq, volar lunotriquetral ligament; RSC, radioscaphocapitate ligament; SC, scaphocapitate ligament.

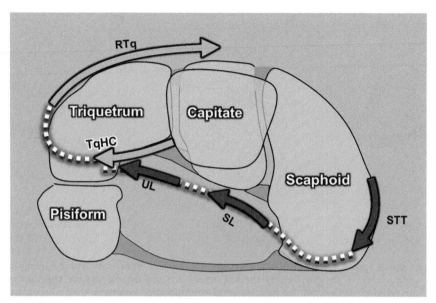

Fig. 6. Ligaments that constrain intracarpal supination. Arranged as a helicoid around the central column, there are 2 groups of ligaments: the medial helicoid antisupination ligaments (*yellow arrows*) and the lateral HASLs (*red arrows*). RTq, dorsal radiotriquetral ligament; SL, scapholunate ligament; STT, scaphotrapeziotrapezoidal ligament; TqHC, triquetrohamate-capitate ligament; UL, ulnolunate ligament.

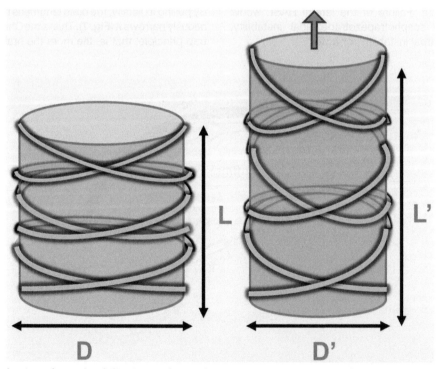

Fig. 7. Mechanism of carpal stabilization under axial traction. Ligaments are set about the wrist as the elastic wires of a Chinese finger trap; that is, like a cylindrical braid made out of helically set ligaments. By pulling it distally, the braid lengthens (L'>L) but simultaneously narrows (D'<D). Based on this principle, the more the wrist is pulled distally, the more compacted are the carpal bones, which are squeezed by the narrowing braid made out of ligaments.

distally, the more the cylinder shrinks, and the forces applied by the trap increase. This mechanism may explain carpal stability under traction.

SUMMARY

Carpal ligaments are not static cable-like collections of fibers holding bones together. Instead they are complex bone-binding structures containing sensorial elements (mechanoreceptors) aiming at detecting changes in carpal bone position and transmitting that information to the sensorimotor system for a centralized control of wrist stability.

Some carpal ligaments are particularly set to detect intracarpal pronation torques. They have been classified as the so-called HAPLs. They are predominately active when the carpus is axially loaded, from distal to proximal, along the longitudinal axis of the hand, or when the distal row is torqued into pronation. The HAPLs play an important role in preventing carpal collapse in patients with chronic scapholunate instability.

The so-called HASLs are formed by ligaments that are only active when the wrist is pulled distally or when the distal row is subjected to a supination torque. They may be subclassified into medial and lateral HASLs. The medial HASL prevents ulnar midcarpal instabilities, whereas the lateral HASL is active in preventing ulnocarpal and lateral midcarpal instability.

REFERENCES

1. Green DP. The 'sprained wrist'. Am Fam Physician 1979;19:114–22.
2. Dobyns JH, Linscheid RL. A short history of the wrist joint. Hand Clin 1997;13:1–12.
3. Jones WA. Beware the sprained wrist. The incidence and diagnosis of scapholunate instability. J Bone Joint Surg Br 1988;70:293–7.
4. Fisk GR. Carpal instability and the fractured scaphoid. Ann R Coll Surg Engl 1970;46:63–76.
5. Linscheid RL, Dobyns JH, Beabout JW, et al. Traumatic instability of the wrist. diagnosis, classification, and pathomechanics. J Bone Joint Surg Am 1972; 54A:1612–32.
6. Dobyns JH, Linscheid RL, Chao EY. Traumatic instability of the wrist. Instr Course Lect 1975;24:189–99.
7. Blatt G. Capsulodesis in reconstructive hand surgery. Dorsal capsulodesis for the unstable scaphoid and volar capsulodesis following excision of the distal ulna. Hand Clin 1987;3:81–102.
8. Watson HK, Ryu J, Akelman E. Limited triscaphoid intercarpal arthrodesis for rotatory subluxation of the scaphoid. J Bone Joint Surg Am 1986;68:345–9.
9. Lavernia CJ, Cohen MS, Taleisnik J. Treatment of scapholunate dissociation by ligamentous repair and capsulodesis. J Hand Surg Am 1992;17: 354–9.
10. Linscheid RL, Dobyns JH. Treatment of scapholunate dissociation. Rotatory subluxation of the scaphoid. Hand Clin 1992;8:645–52.
11. Brunelli GA, Brunelli GR. A new technique to correct carpal instability with scaphoid rotary subluxation: a preliminary report. J Hand Surg Am 1995;20:S82–5.
12. Weiss AP. Scapholunate ligament reconstruction using a bone-retinaculum–bone autograft. J Hand Surg Am 1998;23:205–15.
13. Watson HK, Weinzweig J, Zeppieri J. The natural progression of scaphoid instability. Hand Clin 1997;13:39–49.
14. Linscheid RL, Dobyns JH. Dynamic carpal stability. Keio J Med 2002;51:140–7.
15. Szabo RM. Scapholunate ligament repair with capsulodesis reinforcement. J Hand Surg Am 2008;33: 1645–54.
16. Garcia-Elias M, Lluch AL, Stanley JK. Three-ligament tenodesis for the treatment of scapholunate dissociation: indications and surgical technique. J Hand Surg Am 2006;31:125–34.
17. Bleuler P, Shafighi M, Donati OF, et al. Dynamic repair of scapholunate dissociation with dorsal extensor carpi radialis longus tenodesis. J Hand Surg Am 2008;33:281–4.
18. Wahegaonkar AL, Mathoulin CL. Arthroscopic dorsal capsulo-ligamentous repair in the treatment of chronic scapho-lunate ligament tears. J Wrist Surg 2013;2:141–8.
19. Ross M, Loveridge J, Cutbush K, et al. Scapholunate ligament reconstruction. J Wrist Surg 2013;2:110–5.
20. Corella F, Del Cerro M, Larrainzar-Garijo R, et al. Arthroscopic ligamentoplasty (bone–tendon-tenodesis). A new surgical technique for scapholunate instability: preliminary cadaver study. J Hand Surg Eur Vol 2011;36:682–9.
21. Chee KG, Chin AYH, Chew EM, et al. Antipronation spiral tenodesis - a surgical technique for the treatment of perilunate instabliity. J Hand Surg Am 2012;37:2611–8.
22. Gajendran VK, Peterson B, Slater RR Jr, et al. Long-term outcomes of dorsal intercarpal ligament capsulodesis for chronic scapholunate dissociation. J Hand Surg Am 2007;32:1323–33.
23. Pauchard N, Dederichs A, Segret J, et al. The role of three-ligament tenodesis in the treatment of chronic scapholunate instability. J Hand Surg Eur 2013;38: 758–66.
24. Picha BM, Konstantakos EK, Gordon DA. Incidence of bilateral scapholunate dissociation in symptomatic and asymptomatic wrists. J Hand Surg Am 2012;37:1130–5.
25. Kuo CE, Wolfe SW. Scapholunate instability: current concepts in diagnosis and management. J Hand Surg Am 2008;33:998–1013.

26. Garcia-Elias M, Lluch AL. Wrist instabilities, misalignments and dislocations. In: Wolfe S, Pederson W, Hotchkiss R, et al, editors. Green's operative hand surgery. 7th edition. Atlanta (GA): Elsevier Health Science; 2016. p. 418–78.

27. Riemann BL, Lephart SM. The sensorimotor system, part I: the physiologic basis of functional joint stability. J Athl Train 2002;37:71–9.

28. Hagert E. Proprioception of the wrist joint: a review of current concepts and possible implications on the rehabilitation of the wrist. J Hand Ther 2010;23:2–17.

29. Salva-Coll G, Garcia-Elias M, Hagert E. Scapholunate instability: proprioception and neuromuscular control. J Wrist Surg 2013;2:136–40.

30. Hagert E, Lluch A, Rein S. The role of proprioception and neuromuscular stability in carpal instabilities. J Hand Surg Eur Vol 2016;41:94–101.

31. Esplugas M, Garcia-Elias M, Lluch A, et al. Role of muscles in the stabilization of ligament-deficient wrists. J Hand Ther 2016;29:166–74.

32. Berger RA. The ligaments of the wrist. A current overview of anatomy with considerations of their potential functions. Hand Clin 1997;13:63–82.

33. Sokolow C, Saffar P. Anatomy and histology of the scapholunate ligament. Hand Clin 2001;17:77–81.

34. Frank CB. Ligament structure, physiology and function. J Musculoskelet Neuronal Interact 2004;4: 199–201.

35. Hagert E, Garcia-Elias M, Forsgren S, et al. Immunohistochemical analysis of wrist ligament innervation in relation to their structural composition. J Hand Surg Am 2007;32:30–6.

36. Hagert E, Forsgren S, Ljung BO. Differences in the presence of mechanoreceptors and nerve structures between wrist ligaments may imply differential roles in wrist stabilization. J Orthop Res 2005;23: 757–63.

37. Feipel V, Rooze M. The capsular ligaments of the wrist: morphology, morphometry and clinical applications. Surg Radiol Anat 1999;21:175–80.

38. Garcia-Elias M. Kinetic analysis of carpal stability during grip. Hand Clin 1997;13:151–8.

39. Kobayashi M, Garcia-Elias M, Nagy L, et al. Axial loading induces rotation of the proximal carpal row bones around unique screw-displacement axes. J Biomech 1997;30:1165–7.

Current European Practice in Wrist Arthroplasty

Michel E.H. Boeckstyns, MD, PhD[a],*,
Guillaume Herzberg, MD, PhD[b]

KEYWORDS

- Wrist • Arthroplasty • Prosthesis • Replacement • Arthritis • Joint replacement

KEY POINTS

- Wrist arthroplasty provides functional mobility, improved strength and upper limb function, and reduced pain in carefully selected cases of severely destroyed wrist joints.
- Indications are severe wrist destruction due to rheumatoid arthritis (RA), idiopathic osteoarthritis (OA), scapholunate advanced collapse (SLAC) wrist, malunited intra-articular distal radius fractures, acute irreparable distal radius fractures in the elderly, and Kienböck disease.
- High physical demand, young age, poor bone stock, and spontaneously fused wrist in patients with RA are generally contraindications.
- Implant survival rates have improved with the latest designs but do not compare with the survival rates of hip and knee arthroplasties.

INTRODUCTION

Wrist arthroplasty is still a controversial issue but it has become a challenge to total—and some-times also partial—wrist arthrodesis. The German physician and surgeon, Themistocles Gluck (1853–1942), is said to have performed the first total wrist arthroplasty (TWA) in 1891, using an ivory ball-and-socket device for tuberculosis.[1] At a follow-up of this patient for more than 1 year, the implant was still in place with a good range of motion, but a chronic fistula was present due to the original disease process. He made no further attempts and the idea of wrist arthroplasty using artificial materials was abandoned until John Niebauer[2] and Alfred Swanson[3], during the 1960s, independently introduced the concept of a silicone interpositional spacer for joint replacement that could offer immediate stability and a foundation around which fibrous tissue could grow without inhibiting motion. Swanson started using these silicone implants for the radiocarpal joint in 1967 and reported with his colleagues he reported the long term results in 1984.[3] The results were generally favorable in low-demand rheumatoid patients in the short term,[4] but the silicone spacers are no longer in use for wrist replacement due to problems with breakage, subsidence, and, less frequently, silicone synovitis.[5]

The second generation of implants, introduced in the 1970s, were hard bearing multicomponent implants.[6–10] There is no consensus on the definition of second-generation implants but they generally consist of a radial component and a carpal component that is fixed into 1 or more of the metacarpal bones after wide bone resection. Many second-generation implants turned out

The authors have nothing to disclose.
[a] CFR Hospitals, Hans Bekkevold Alle 2b, Hellerup 2900, Denmark; [b] Unit of Wrist Surgery, Edouard Heriot Hospital, 5 Place d'Arsonval, Lyon 69003, France
* Corresponding author.
E-mail address: mibo@dadlnet.dk

hand.theclinics.com

to have unsatisfactory long-term results; they are no longer available. The published series are generally small and with short follow-up. The most well documented is the Biax (DePuy, Warsaw, Indiana), which was withdrawn from the market for commercial reasons.[11]

The third generation of TWA (sometimes called the fourth generation) is the currently available implants; they are characterized by moderate bone resection and avoid fixation in the metacarpal bones, with the exception of an optional, short length of screw fixation in the index finger metacarpal (**Fig. 1**). They attempt to mimic the natural anatomy and biomechanics of the wrist and are largely unconstrained.[12–14] The commonly used implants in Europe are the Universal2 (Integra, Plainsboro, New Jersey), the ReMotion (Stryker, Kalamazoo, Michigan), and the Maestro (Biomet, Warsaw, Indiana). In recent years, the French Amandys (Tornier [Bioprofile], Grenoble, France) was introduced as a single-component pyrocarbon interposition arthroplasty.[15] Pyrocarbon can also be used to replace the head of the capitate combined with a proximal row carpectomy.[16] Another recent European design is the Motec (Swemac, Linköping, Sweden), which differs from the other currently available implants by being metal-on-metal and fixed with large screws in the radius and the long (middle) finger metacarpal.[17] Hemiarthroplasties, using the radial component of third-generation implants or special radial implants, are also used[18–22] in the French Prosthelast (Agro-médical, Cham, Switzerland)[23] and Roux (now: SOPHIA, Biotech, Paris, France)[19] prostheses.

INDICATIONS AND CONTRAINDICATIONS

In general, the indication for wrist replacement is a severely destroyed and painful wrist in which conservative means have not provided adequate pain relief and in which other motion-preserving procedures are impossible, hopeless, or have failed. For several decades, the main indication was RA. Since the turn of the century, however, other conditions have increasingly been of interest.[11] Today, the debate over indications is polarized between the rheumatoid wrist, generally in low-demand patients but with poorer bone stock, and idiopathic or posttraumatic OA—those patients generally have better bone stock but are also more physically active. There is no clear evidence about which indications lead to the best results and the fewest complications: it seems that carefully selected patients with RA or OA do equally well.[24] For patients with SLAC III wrist, other interventions may be considered, such as a 4-corner fusion. It is to some extent a subjective evaluation that can be influenced by previous experience with other motion-preserving procedures. In cases of an irreparable joint surface of the distal radius in elderly low-demand patients with an intra-articular distal radius fracture, hemiarthroplasty (HA) may be a solution.[20,22]

Box 1 summarizes the authors' views on factors in favor of TWA versus a total wrist fusion when advising patients needing a surgical procedure for painful panarthritis of the wrist. These factors must be considered in combination with each other; none of them is decisive considered alone. Younger patients less than or equal to 50 year old—implying an active lifestyle and a long life expectancy—and severely osteoporotic or destroyed bone stock are the main contraindications to wrist arthroplasty. Wrists with very poor

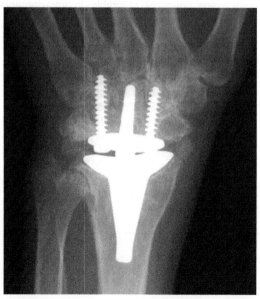

Fig. 1. ReMotion TWA in a rheumatoid patient. (*Courtesy of* Stryker, Kalamazoo, Michigan.)

Box 1
Factors in favor of wrist arthroplasty

- Functional wrist motion
- Elderly patient
- Low physical work load
- Low physical loading in leisure activities
- Poor function of the contralateral wrist (incl. wrist fusion)
- Poor shoulder, elbow, or finger function
- Good bone stock and quality
- No severe radiocarpal instability
- Expected good compliance with therapy and advice about care of the implant

motion, for example, a spontaneously fused rheumatoid wrist of Simmen type I,[25] are generally considered a contraindication to wrist arthroplasty, because restoration of a useful mobility cannot be expected in these cases. On the other hand, poor function of other joints that could compensate for stiffness of the wrist or that benefit from some wrist motion, like the metacarpophalangeal joints of the fingers in patients with RA, favor arthroplasty rather than fusion.

SURGICAL TECHNIQUE

Wrist arthroplasty requires a high level of expertise. It may be performed under general anesthesia or regional block. In cases of a regional block, techniques that reduce imbalance in the muscular control of the shoulder must be used to avoid excessive external rotation of the arm during surgery. Day surgery may be considered if adequate postoperative pain control can be offered to patients; this requires a high degree of compliance. If possible, postoperative administration of a local anesthetic like lignocaine by an axillary catheter can be useful, in combination with oral analgesics. A tourniquet time of approximately 2 hours must be expected for total arthroplasty and 1 hour for hemiarthroplasty or interpositional arthroplasty.

The wrist is approached through a dorsal midline incision. The extensor retinaculum is divided according to surgeon preference; most surgeons use an incision that offers the possibility of lengthening the retinaculum, using it to reinforce the joint capsule or interposing the tissue between the extensor tendons and the implant if needed. Most implants require a large capsular opening rather than a ligament-sparing opening. In patients with concomitant distal radioulnar joint problems, the authors advise a simple resection of the ulnar head (Darrach procedure) rather than an ulnar head replacement; there is no evidence that a more demanding procedure on top of a complicated index procedure offers any advantage. Guides to perform the bony resections are usually available. It is advisable to fuse the remaining carpal bones. After the introduction of the latest generation of implants, an uncemented technique is used by most surgeons, except in very osteoporotic bone. Pyrocarbon interpositional implants are not fixed into bone.[15] Intraoperative image intensifier control is mandatory. Usually some kind of postoperative motion restriction is applied during the first 2 weeks to 3 weeks and loaded mobilization is initiated only after a minimum of 6 weeks postoperatively.

COMPLICATIONS
General Complications

The rate of deep postoperative infections is reported to be very low with the use of the latest-generation implants.[11] Instability with dislocation was frequent with the first version of the Universal Wrist (KMI, Carlsbad, California), up to 14%,[12,26] but this problem seems largely to have been solved with the modified version, the Universal2[18,27,28] and has not been a major problem with other newer designs.[11] In the systematic review from 2009 to 2013 by Yeoh and Tourret,[29] a detailed analysis of minor and major complications reported in the literature is listed: wound problems, 3% to 17%; instability, 4%; superficial infection, 4.7% to 14%; deep infection, 3% to 4%; synovitis, 4%; scar sensitivity, 9.5%; reduced range of motion, 9.5% to 22%; tendon laceration/rupture, 3% to 4.7%; periprosthetic fracture, 4.6%; nerve problems, 3% to 9%; dislocations, 21.8%; nonunion of the arthrodesis, 10%; and impingement and need of further surgery to the distal ulna, 16.7%. Gaspar and colleagues[29] reported a high number of minor complications after the Maestro and after hemiarthroplasty.

Periprosthetic Osteolysis

Aseptic periprosthetic osteolysis (PPO) after second-generation or third-generation TWA, with or without frank loosening of the implant components has previously been reported in the literature but rarely in a systematic way.[8,9,17,24,26,28,31–41] It may be associated with gross loosening of the prosthetic components but this is not always the case.[17,24,28,31,34,36,38,39,42] The cause of osteolysis is not evident. Polyethylene-induced osteolysis has been considered but this does not explain why the phenomenon also encountered with metal-on-metal implants.[17,41] There seems not to be a direct correlation between the magnitude of osteolysis and the amount of polyethylene or metallic debris in samples taken from the implant bone interface.[43] Besides the host response to particulate debris, early micromotion before bone ingrowth, high interfacial shear stress, high fluid pressure, damage to blood vessels, and stress shielding have all been considered, but so far the exact pathophysiology of the osteolysis remains an enigma. In the vast majority of cases, the radiologic radiolucent zones of PPO are confined to the peri-implant margins; they are usually less than 2 mm wide. They may increase in as much as 15% of cases, however, but tend to stabilize after a few years[42] **(Fig. 2)**. Regardless of the mechanism, PPO constitutes a risk factor for prosthetic loosening, mainly the carpal components. There

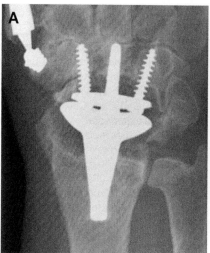 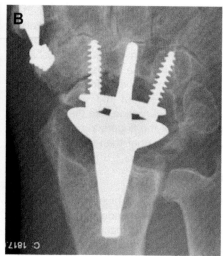

Fig. 2. PPO 4 years and 6 years after cementless implantation of a ReMotion TWA in a rheumatoid patient.(*A*) is 4 years after operation. (*B*) is 6 years after operation. (*Courtesy of* Stryker, Kalamazoo, Michigan.)

are different opinions concerning the treatment strategy in case of marked asymptomatic PPO; some investigators advise revision of the implants, which also could imply conversion to total wrist fusion[26] and some investigators advise curettage and bone grafting, whereas others choose an expectant attitude with close observation.[42]

OUTCOMES

In general, the mean values for ranges of motion at follow-up are similar for most implants and generally close to the functional range defined by Palmer and colleagues,[44] although somewhat smaller than the more rigorous range defined by Ryu and colleagues.[45] Most series report a mean postoperative range of flexion-extension of approximately 60° to 70° and a range of radoulnar deviation of 25° to 30°.[11] An exception is the Maestro, which may yield better ranges of motion.[14,46] The change in motion from before operation to follow-up is not

consistent, but generally TWA does not result in an appreciably improved motion.

In a published series in which patient-rated outcome measures were recorded preoperatively and postoperatively, improvement in scores was reported (**Table 1**). In most patients, pain reduces and grip strength increases.[11,29]

Implant Survival, Prosthetic Loosening, and Revision Surgery

The reported survival of third-generation TWA implants varies markedly from one publication to another. It ranges from 100% with a mean follow-up period of 5.5 years[28] to 62% at 8 years.[26] Most series report a cumulative implant survival at 5 years to 8 years of approximately 90% or greater[24,46–48] (**Fig. 3**). Survival curves of the Kaplan-Meier type, however, do not reflect the true rate of loosening; some of the surviving implants may be clinically well tolerated but radiologically loose.[47]

Table 1
Functional improvement after total wrist arthroplasty–evaluated with patient-rated outcome measures

Series	Patient-rated Outcome Measure	Mean Improvement in Patient-rated Outcome Measures Score (Points)
Herzberg, 2012[24]	QuickDASH	20
van Winterswijk, 2010[53]	DASH	24
Ward, 2011[26]	DASH	22
Morapudi, 2012[27]	DASH	10
	PRWE	46

Abbreviations: DASH, disabilities of the arm, shoulder, and hand questionnaire; PRWE, patient-rated wrist evaluation questionnaire.

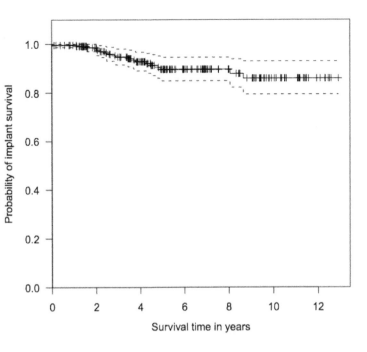

Fig. 3. Updated cumulated survival curve for the ReMotion TWA. (*Courtesy of* Stryker, Kalamazoo, MI; and *Data from* The international [European] wrist arthroplasty register. Available at: https://stacom.dk/irwa. Accessed November 5, 2016; with permission.)

In the vast majority of failures, the cause is loosening of the carpal component (**Fig. 4**). This has led to the concept of HA, using a radial implant in combination with a proximal row carpectomy. The indications have been arthritic changes after distal radius fractures or severe SLAC deformity rather than RA.[18,30] HA has also been used as a primary solution for irreparable distal radius fractures in elderly patients.[19,20,22,23] Only short-term follow-up studies are available,[18,21,30] making it

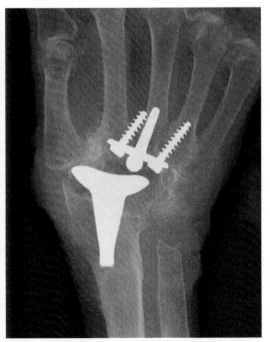

Fig. 4. Loosened carpal component of a ReMotion TWA 6 years after implantation in a rheumatoid patient. (*Courtesy of* Stryker, Kalamazoo, Michigan.)

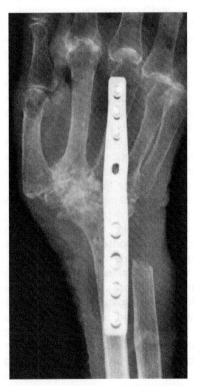

Fig. 5. Same case as in **Fig. 4** after revision to a total wrist fusion.

impossible to compare HA with TWA. Although HA seems straightforward, it is not always so.

The pyrocarbon interposition arthroplasty is a different concept. It consists of a quadric elliptical spacer that is not fixed to the bones. Bone resection is similar to the resection needed for the latest TWAs but a ligament-sparing technique can be used. Long-term results have not been published but the results in the short term seem promising. Because there is almost certainly some concommittant carpal instability and the implant cannot correct that, it is inevitable that the implant is unstable initially, although it may stabilize through scar tissue.[49]

Although a failed TWA of the latest generation may be revised to a new TWA, total wrist arthrodesis with a bone graft remains the most common salvage procedure.[50–52] This is usually stabilized with a plate and screws (**Fig. 5**). This is often a complex procedure.

FUTURE PERSPECTIVES

Wrist arthroplasty has increasingly become a challenge to total wrist arthrodesis. The results are generally good for pain relief, increased grip strength, and improved upper limb function. Motion is preserved but does not usually improve on the preoperative range of motion. The rate of perioperative and postoperative complications may be high.

In the twenty-first century, indications have gradually moved from low-demand patients with RA to other conditions, such as idiopathic OA, SLAC wrist, malunited distal radius fractures, Kienböck disease, and so forth. The survival of the currently available third-generation implants seems better than was obtained with earlier designs.

One of the major concerns after TWA is development of periprosthetic osteolysis. So far the pathophysiology of the osteolysis remains an enigma but it is a risk factor for later mechanical failure, especially the carpal component of most designs. There are still significant problems with carpal component loosening; some surviving implants are radiologically loose at long-term follow-up, although clinically tolerated. Thus, there is a need to continuously strive at improve prosthetic designs and surgical skills. Patient selection probably plays a major role. Recent concepts (HA and pyrocarbon interpositional arthroplasty) have been aimed at reducing carpal component loosening, but only short-term results of small series have been published. One newer design—the Motec—has returned to metacarpal fixation.

Providing patients with correct information regarding the results and the complications of wrist arthroplasty, discussing the pros and the cons of arthroplasty and arthrodesis, and at the same time selecting patients for one or the other procedure is still a complex task, requiring considerable expertise and experience.

REFERENCES

1. Ritt MJ, Stuart PR, Naggar L, et al. The early history of arthroplasty of the wrist. From amputation to total wrist implant. J Hand Surg Am 1994;19:778–82.
2. Niebauer JJ, Shaw JL, Doren WW. Silicone-dacron hinge prosthesis. Design, evaluation, and application. Ann Rheum Dis 1969;28(Suppl 5): 56–8.
3. Swanson AB, de Groot Swanson G, Maupin BK. Flexible implant arthroplasty of the radiocarpal joint. Surgical technique and long-term study. Clin Orthop Relat Res 1984;(187):94–106.
4. Lundkvist L, Barfred T. Total wrist arthroplasty. Experience with swanson flexible silicone implants, 1982-1988. Scand J Plast Reconstr Surg Hand Surg 1992; 26:97–100.
5. Schill S, Thabe H, Mohr W. [Long-term outcome of Swanson prosthesis management of the rheumatic wrist joint]. Handchir Mikrochir Plast Chir 2001;33: 198–206 [in German].
6. Cobb TK, Beckenbaugh RD. Biaxial total-wrist arthroplasty. J Hand Surg Am 1996;21:1011–21.
7. Meuli HC. Arthroplasty of the wrist. Clin Orthop Relat Res 1980;149:118–25.
8. Rahimtoola ZO, Rozing PM. Preliminary results of total wrist arthroplasty using the RWS Prosthesis. J Hand Surg Br 2003;28:54–60.
9. Rahimtoola ZO, Hubach P. Total modular wrist prosthesis: a new design. Scand J Plast Reconstr Surg Hand Surg 2004;38:160–5.
10. Volz RG. The development of a total wrist arthroplasty. Clin Orthop Relat Res 1976;116:209–14.
11. Boeckstyns ME. Wrist arthroplasty–a systematic review. Dan Med J 2014;61:A4834.
12. Menon J. Universal total wrist implant: experience with a carpal component fixed with three screws. J Arthroplasty 1998;13:515–23.
13. Herzberg G. Prospective study of a new total wrist arthroplasty: short term results. Chir Main 2011;30: 20–5.
14. Nydick JA, Greenberg SM, Stone JD, et al. Clinical outcomes of total wrist arthroplasty. J Hand Surg Am 2012;37:1580–4.
15. Bellemere P, Maes-Clavier C, Loubersac T, et al. Amandys((R)) implant: novel pyrocarbon arthroplasty for the wrist. Chir Main 2012;31:176–87.
16. Szalay G, Stigler B, Kraus R, et al. [Proximal row carpectomy and replacement of the proximal pole of the capitate by means of a pyrocarbon cap (RCPI)

in advanced carpal collapse]. Handchir Mikrochir Plast Chir 2012;44:17–22.

17. Reigstad O, Lutken T, Grimsgaard C, et al. Promising one- to six-year results with the Motec wrist arthroplasty in patients with post-traumatic osteoarthritis. J Bone Joint Surg Br 2012;94:1540–5.

18. Adams BD. Wrist arthroplasty: partial and total. Hand Clin 2013;29:79–89.

19. Roux JL. [Replacement and resurfacing prosthesis of the distal radius: a new therapeutic concept]. Chir Main 2009;28:10–7.

20. Vergnenegre G, Hardy J, Mabit C, et al. Hemiarthroplasty for complex distal radius fractures in elderly patients. J Wrist Surg 2015;4:169–73.

21. Culp RW, Bachoura A, Gelman SE, et al. Proximal row carpectomy combined with wrist hemiarthroplasty. J Wrist Surg 2012;1:39–46.

22. Herzberg G, Burnier M, Marc A, et al. Primary wrist hemiarthroplasty for irreparable distal radius fracture in the independent elderly. J Wrist Surg 2015; 4:156–63.

23. Ichihara S, Diaz JJ, Peterson B, et al. Distal radius isoelastic resurfacing prosthesis: a preliminary report. J Wrist Surg 2015;4:150–5.

24. Herzberg G, Boeckstyns M, Sorensen AL, et al. "Remotion" total wrist arthroplasty: preliminary results of a prospective international multicenter study of 215 cases. J Wrist Surg 2012;1:17–22.

25. Simmen BR, Huber H. [The wrist joint in chronic polyarthritis–a new classification based on the type of destruction in relation to the natural course and the consequences for surgical therapy]. Handchir Mikrochir Plast Chir 1994;26: 182–9.

26. Ward CM, Kuhl T, Adams BD. Five to ten-year outcomes of the Universal total wrist arthroplasty in patients with rheumatoid arthritis. J Bone Joint Surg Am 2011;93:914–9.

27. Morapudi SP, Marlow WJ, Withers D, et al. Total wrist arthroplasty using the Universal 2 prosthesis. J Orthop Surg 2012;20:365–8.

28. Ferreres A, Lluch A, Del Valle M. Universal total wrist arthroplasty: midterm follow-up study. J Hand Surg Am 2011;36:967–73.

29. Yeoh D, Tourret L. Total wrist arthroplasty: a systematic review of the evidence from the last five years. J Hand Surg Eur Vol 2015;40:458–68.

30. Gaspar MP, Lou J, Kane PM, et al. Complications following partial and total wrist arthroplasty: a single-center retrospective review. J Hand Surg Am 2016;41:47–53.e4.

31. Lirette R, Kinnard P. Biaxial total wrist arthroplasty in rheumatoid arthritis. Can J Surg 1995;38:51–3.

32. Stegeman M, Rijnberg WJ, van Loon CJ. Biaxial total wrist arthroplasty in rheumatoid arthritis. Satisfactory functional results. Rheumatol Int 2005;25: 191–4.

33. Courtman NH, Sochart DH, Trail IA, et al. Biaxial wrist replacement. Initial results in the rheumatoid patient. J Hand Surg Br 1999;24:32–4.

34. Harlingen D, Heesterbeek PJ, J de Vos M. High rate of complications and radiographic loosening of the biaxial total wrist arthroplasty in rheumatoid arthritis: 32 wrists followed for 6 (5-8) years. Acta Orthop 2011;82:721–6.

35. Kretschmer F, Fansa H. [BIAX total wrist arthroplasty: management and results after 42 patients]. Handchir Mikrochir Plast Chir 2007;39:238–48.

36. Rizzo M, Beckenbaugh RD. Results of biaxial total wrist arthroplasty with a modified (long) metacarpal stem. J Hand Surg Am 2003;28:577–84.

37. Fourastier J, Le Breton L, Alnot Y, et al. [Guepar's total radio-carpal prosthesis in the surgery of the rheumatoid wrist. Apropos of 72 cases reviewed]. Rev Chir Orthop Reparatrice Appar Mot 1996;82: 108–15 [in French].

38. Bidwai AS, Cashin F, Richards A, et al. Short to medium results using the remotion total wrist replacement for rheumatoid arthritis. Hand Surg 2013;18:175–8.

39. Gellman H, Hontas R, Brumfield RH Jr, et al. Total wrist arthroplasty in rheumatoid arthritis. A long-term clinical review. Clin Orthop Relat Res 1997; 342:71–6.

40. Bosco JA 3rd, Bynum DK, Bowers WH. Long-term outcome of Volz total wrist arthroplasties. J Arthroplasty 1994;9:25–31.

41. Radmer S, Andresen R, Sparmann M. Total wrist arthroplasty in patients with rheumatoid arthritis. J Hand Surg Am 2003;28:789–94.

42. Boeckstyns MEH, Herzberg G. Periprosthetic osteolysis after total wrist arthroplasty. J Wrist Surg 2014;3:101–6.

43. Boeckstyns ME, Toxvaerd A, Bansal M, et al. Wear particles and osteolysis in patients with total wrist arthroplasty. J Hand Surg Am 2014;39: 2396–404.

44. Palmer AK, Werner FW, Murphy D, et al. Functional wrist motion: a biomechanical study. J Hand Surg Am 1985;10:39–46.

45. Ryu JY, Cooney WP 3rd, Askew LJ, et al. Functional ranges of motion of the wrist joint. J Hand Surg Am 1991;16:409–19.

46. Sagerfors M, Gupta A, Brus O, et al. Patient related functional outcome after total wrist arthroplasty: a single center study of 206 cases. Hand Surg 2015; 20:81–7.

47. Boeckstyns ME, Herzberg G, Merser S. Favorable results after total wrist arthroplasty: 65 wrists in 60 patients followed for 5-9 years. Acta Orthop 2013; 84:415–9.

48. Reigstad A, Mjorud J. Results of 189 wrist replacements. Acta Orthop 2012;83:101.

49. Giddins G. Editorial. J Hand Surg Eur Vol 2012; 37:489.

50. Adams BD, Kleinhenz BP, Guan JJ. Wrist arthrodesis for failed total wrist arthroplasty. J Hand Surg Eur Vol 2017;42:84–9.

51. Reigstad O, Holm-Glad T, Thorkildsen R, et al. Successful conversion of wrist prosthesis to arthrodesis in 11 patients. J Hand Surg Eur Vol 2016. [Epub ahead of print].

52. Rizzo M, Ackerman DB, Rodrigues RL, et al. Wrist arthrodesis as a salvage procedure for failed implant arthroplasty. J Hand Surg Eur Vol 2011;36:29–33.

53. van Winterswijk PJ, Bakx PA. Promising clinical results of the universal total wrist prosthesis in rheumatoid arthritis. Open Orthop J 2010;4:67–70.

Treatment of Intra-articular Distal Radius Fractures

Shohei Omokawa, MD, PhD[a],*, Yukio Abe, MD, PhD[b],
Junya Imatani, MD, PhD[c], Hisao Moritomo, MD, PhD[d],
Daisuke Suzuki, MD[e], Tadanobu Onishi, MD[f]

KEYWORDS

- Intra-articular distal radius fracture • Arthroscopy • Fracture malunion
- Triangular fibrocartilage complex • Scapholunate ligament • Distal radioulnar joint

KEY POINTS

- Understanding of detailed morphology of the distal radius is required to prevent flexor tendon problems after plate surgery.
- A plate presetting and arthroscopic reduction technique (PART) is described, that can simplify combination of plating and arthroscopy in treating this fracture.
- Complete ligament rupture at dorsal scapholunate ligament (SL) space and foveal triangular fibrocartilage complex (TFCC) attachment can be diagnosed arthroscopically, and the repair may lead to better clinical results rather than attempting to manage chronic instability.
- Accurate corrective osteotomy for intra-articular fracture malunion is possible using CT bone models and a custom-made surgical template.

DISTAL RADIUS MORPHOLOGY

Volar locking plate (VLP) fixation is popular in the treatment of unstable distal radius fractures (DRFs). In surgical management of DRFs with severe comminution or marked osteoporosis, the authors believe it is particularly important to apply a subchondral buttress fixation involving distal locking screws and a plate to stabilize the volar fragment. In these cases, very distal placement of the locking plate may be necessary[1] but with a risk of flexor tendon impingement.

The Watershed Line Revisited

Orbay[2] reported that the concave surface of the volar radius was limited distally by a transverse ridge or watershed line. Implants placed over or projecting above the watershed line can potentially irritate and even lead to the rupture of the flexor tendons.

The authors recorded the macroscopic appearance of the volar aspect of the distal radius, volar radiocarpal ligaments, and pronator quadratus.[3] Ulnarly the volar radius had 2 main distal transverse lines indicating the bony prominence. One

Disclosure Statement: The authors have nothing to disclose.
[a] Department of Hand Surgery, Nara Medical University, 840 Shijyo-cho, Kashihara, Nara 634-8521, Japan;
[b] Department of Orthopaedic Surgery, Saiseikai Shimonoseki General Hospital, 8-5-1 Yasuoka-cho, Shimonoseki, Yamaguchi 759-6603, Japan; [c] Department of Orthopaedic Surgery, Okayama Saiseikai General Hospital, 2-25 Kokutaicho Kita-ku, Okayama, Okayama 700-8511, Japan; [d] Yukioka Hospital Hand Center, Osaka Yukioka College of Health Science, 2-2-3 Ukita, Kita-ku, Osaka, Osaka 530-0021, Japan; [e] Hand Surgery Center, Nishi-Nara Central Hospital, 1-15 Tsurumainishi, Nara, Nara 631-0024, Japan; [f] Department of Orthopaedic Surgery, Nara Medical University, 840 Shijyo-cho, Kashihara, Nara 634-8521, Japan
* Corresponding author.
E-mail address: omokawa@gaia.eonet.ne.jp

Hand Clin 33 (2017) 529–543
http://dx.doi.org/10.1016/j.hcl.2017.04.009
0749-0712/17/© 2017 Elsevier Inc. All rights reserved.

comprises the distal higher bony prominent line and the other comprises the proximal lower bony prominent line forming the distal bony ridge of the pronator fossa (**Fig. 1**). Radially these 2 lines merge. The volar radius also has radial and ulnar bony prominences (see **Fig. 1**; **Fig. 2**) on the distal higher line, which can be palpated in all specimens even on the articular capsule and volar radiocarpal ligaments. The ulnar bony prominence is larger than the radial bony prominence and the highest point on the volar aspect of the distal end of the radius. A line connecting the distal margin of the pronator quadratus (see **Fig. 1**) does not correspond to the distal ridge of the pronator fossa.

Another study by the authors showed that the flexor digitorum profundus (FDP) tendon of the index finger runs on the radial surface of the ulnar bony prominence. The flexor pollicis longus (FPL) tendon runs just laterally to the FDP tendon in all 26 specimens.[4] Therefore, the ulnar bony prominence on the volar aspect of the distal end of the radius is a reliable landmark. The dangerous zone for flexor impingement was a mean of 11 mm ± 1 mm radial to the ulnar bony prominence of the volar distal end of the radius in the 26 specimens. In this zone, surgeons should avoid volar implants protruding anterior to the volar rim

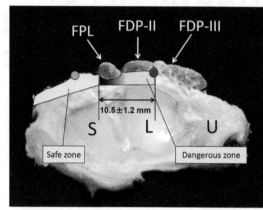

Fig. 2. Articular view. The radial prominence is indicated by the blue dot and the ulnar prominence by the red dot. The FDP tendon to the index finger runs on the lateral surface of the ulnar prominence. The FPL tendon runs just laterally to the FDP II and III tendon of the index and middle finger and between the 2 bony prominences in all specimens. The dangerous zone is 10 mm ± 1 mm radial to the ulnar prominence of the radius. In this zone, the volar implants should not be projected anterior to the rim of the distal radius. L, lunate bone; S, scaphoid bone; U, ulna.

of the distal radius (see **Fig. 2**). Microscopically, the authors assessed a series of sagittal sections of the wrist regions to investigate the positional relationships over the volar aspect of the distal radius, pronator quadratus, intermediate fibrous zone, and radiocarpal ligaments (**Fig. 3**).

The authors believe that the watershed line is not a distinct line; it corresponds to the distal margin of the pronator fossa in the radial aspect of the volar radius and to a hypothetical line between the distal and proximal lines in the ulnar aspect. The radial and ulnar bony prominences on the volar radius should be key structures for accurate plate placement to avoid flexor tendon injury.

Volar Morphology of the Distal Radius

Based on CT scans of 70 normal forearms, Oura and colleagues[5] found that the concavity depth was at its maximum (1.7 ± 0.8 mm) at 6 mm proximal to the palmar edge of the lunate fossa and progressively decreases toward the proximal radius. The FPL is closest to the radius at 2 mm proximal to the palmar edge of the lunate fossa; the volar surface of the distal radius was supinated from proximal to distal (mean external rotation: 10°). Yoneda and colleagues[6] investigated the teardrop height ratio and teardrop inclination angle, representing the volar projection of the lunate facet of the distal radius; they showed

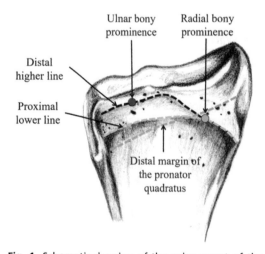

Fig. 1. Schematic drawing of the volar aspect of the radius. The 2 dotted lines indicate the bony inflexion points based on the macroscopic and microscopic observations. The black dotted line indicates the distal higher bony inflexion points, and the yellow dotted line indicates the proximal lower bony inflexion points, as the most distal ridge of the pronator fossa. The green dotted line indicates the distal margin of the pronator quadratus muscle. In addition, there are 2 bony prominences, ulnar and radial, on the black dotted line indicated by the red dot and blue dot, respectively.

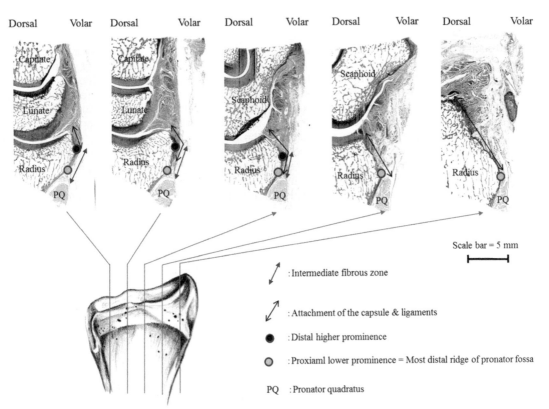

Dorsal Volar Dorsal Volar Dorsal Volar Dorsal Volar Dorsal Volar

Scale bar = 5 mm

↗ : Intermediate fibrous zone

↗ : Attachment of the capsule & ligaments

● : Distal higher prominence

○ : Proxiaml lower prominence = Most distal ridge of pronator fossa

PQ : Pronator quadratus

Fig. 3. Sagittal sections of the distal end of the radius and volar wrist region. The black dots indicate the distal higher prominence. The yellow dots indicate the proximal lower prominence, at the most distal ridge of the pronator fossa. The black arrows indicate the attachment of the volar joint capsule and ligament. The red double arrows indicate the intermediate fibrous zone between the radiocarpal ligament and the pronator quadratus (PQ) muscle. (*Adapted from* Imatani J, Akita K, Yamaquchi K, et al. An anatomic study of the watershed line on the volar, distal aspect of the radius: implications for plate placement and avoidance of tendon ruptures. J Hand Surg Am 2012;37(8):1552; with permission.)

considerable variation in 200 standardized lateral wrist radiographs. They found that the fits of all plates differed significantly between bones, with the radii with the lowest teardrop inclination angle the closest approximation to that of each plate, suggesting that careful plate selection may be necessary. The study of Pichler and colleagues[7] suggests different surface curvatures of the distal radius may lead to plate rotation.

FRACTURES CLASSIFICATION

Several classification systems have described the pattern of intra-articular DRFs[8–11]; CT imaging is more reliable than plain radiographs.[12] An intra-articular fragment often cannot be successfully reduced by ligamentotaxis; loss of reduction may result in unsatisfactory clinical outcomes but is often well tolerated. Trumble and colleagues[9] reported on scaphoid and lunate die punch fragment depression in the scaphoid or lunate fossae; they reported that patients with a fracture at least

1 mm of displacement at the articular surface benefited from open surgical treatment. Medoff[10] reported that intra-articular fragments were almost always associated with axial loading injuries. The magnitude of displacement and the sizes of the intra-articular fragments, however, were not evaluated.

Intra-articular Central Depression Fragment

The authors analyzed 145 consecutive intra-articular fractures using both 3-D and multiplanar reconstruction CT images, focusing on intra-articular central depression fragments, and recorded the location, size, and maximum displacement of each fragment. In addition to centrally located and depressed fragments, displaced sigmoid notch fragments without ligamentous attachment were defined as central depression fragments. The authors expressed the fragment size as the maximum depth (volar to dorsal) and width (ulnar to radial) and measured the maximum displacement as the sum of the gap and step-off by Cole and colleagues' arc method.[13]

Eleven central depression fragments were found in 9 wrists. All the fragments were depressed relative to the marginal fragments; the mean displacement was 3 (range: 0.3–8) mm. There were 4 fragments involving the scaphoid facet only (mean size: 10 mm × 7 mm); 4 lunate facet fragments (mean size: 8 mm × 6 mm); and 3 fragments involved both the scaphoid and lunate facets (mean size: 8 mm × 9 mm). Displacement of scaphoid facet fragments (mean depth: 4.7 mm) was larger than that of lunate facet fragments (1.3 mm). The presence of a central depression fragment had a positive correlation with the number of articular fragments and presence of a volar rim fragment (r = 0.39 and r = 0.34, respectively; p<.001).

Central depression fragments were found in 6% of intra-articular DRFs; they were likely to occur with volar rim fragments in severely comminuted fractures. Because central depression fragments may not move with ligamentotaxis, preoperative recognition and surgical intervention by fluoroscopic or arthroscopic reduction of these fragments, especially scaphoid die punch fragments,[14] may be necessary to minimize the risk of postoperative osteoarthritis.

NOVEL ARTHROSCOPIC TECHNIQUE AND FINDINGS

Wrist arthroscopy is currently believed by some enthusiasts to be an important adjunct procedure in the surgical management of a DRF but it is not proved.[15–17] Wrist arthroscopy becomes troublesome when VLP fixation is conducted, because the vertical traction for arthroscopy needs to be both applied and released during surgery. The authors have developed a plate presetting and arthroscopic reduction techniqiue (PART) that can simplify the combination of plating and arthroscopy.[18,19] The details of the PART are as follows.

Surgical Procedure

Via a standard volar radial approach, the fracture is exposed and reduced by manipulating the fragments. Because the palmar cortex of the radius is generally less comminuted, reduction of the palmar cortex is an indicator of anatomic reduction. Several intrafocal pins are inserted to reduce the metaphyseal alignment radially and dorsally. After an adequate reduction — including the articular surface, if possible — is achieved, the fragments are fixed under fluoroscopy with several percutaneous interfragmentary pins. Four to five 1.5-mm Kirschner's wires (k-wires) are inserted

for a typical intra-articular fracture (**Fig. 4**). Placement of the wires should not interfere with placement of the VLP. The intrafocal pins are important to maintain alignment when arthroscopic reduction of the intra-articular fragments is required, because the interfragmentary pins need to be removed to reduce the intra-articular fragments. After temporary fracture fixation by the K-wires, the locking plate is preset palmarly on the radius and temporarily fixed with a screw inserted into the proximal fragment using the oval hole of the plate, thus allowing slight regulation of the plate placement at the final fixation.

Wrist arthroscopy is performed in vertical traction. The authors generally use 2 dorsal portals to evaluate and treat the intra-articular fragments and soft tissue injuries; the 3-4 and 4-5 portals. In addition, the authors sometimes use a palmar portal through the floor of the FCR tendon to investigate a palmar segment tear of the scapholunate interosseous ligament (SLIL) and dorsal fracture fragments.[20,21] A 2.3-mm arthroscope with a 30° field of vision is introduced through the 3-4 portal and a probe or shaver is inserted through the 4-5 portal. The remaining hematoma in the joint is removed. The joint is inspected thoroughly in particular for fracture fragments and soft tissue injuries.

Fracture fragments that are not reduced by the initial manipulation are now reduced under arthroscopic control. K-wires preventing reduction of a displaced fracture fragment are removed or used for a joystick maneuver. Any central depression can be reduced by pushing up from the intramedullary canal using a probe, inserted at the dorsal or palmar fracture site. Displaced neighboring fracture fragments can be reduced by percutaneous clamping using a tenaculum (**Fig. 5**). Free fracture fragments that are too small to fix are removed using arthroscopic shaver. After reduction of the fracture fragments is achieved, temporary K-wire fixation is performed. These K-wires are removed after insertion of locking screws through the distal plate holes.

The necessity for initial treatment of soft tissue injuries remains controversial. The authors' beliefs are that if an SLIL injury is recognized, midcarpal arthroscopy is performed to evaluate SL stability with a probe. Similarly, if distal radioulnar joint (DRUJ) instability is suspected, DRUJ arthroscopy is performed to confirm a foveal tear of the TFCC. The authors' strategy for treatment of SLIL injuries according to Geissler and colleagues'[22] classification is immobilization of the wrist joint for 4 weeks to 5 weeks for grade III instability, pinning and repair of the dorsal part of the SLIL, and augmentation with some dorsal intercarpal ligament for

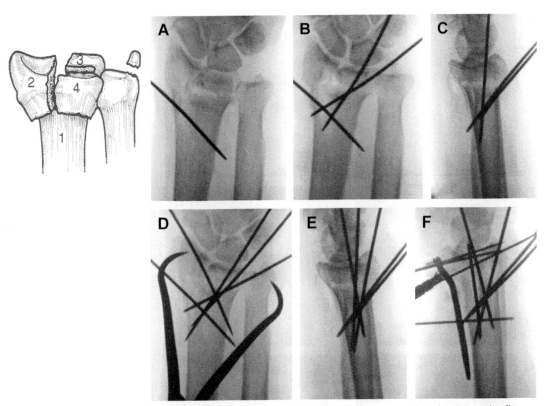

Fig. 4. (*A–F*) Several intrafocal and interfragmental K-wires are inserted to fix anatomic reduction under fluoroscopy (*A–E*) for typical intra-articular fracture. The palmar locking plate is put palmar on the radius and temporarily fixed (*F*). (*A-E*) Indicate sequential reduction procedure by k-wires and clamping.

grade IV instability. For a foveal tear of the TFCC, the authors perform the repair arthroscopically.[23] The authors believe these procedures are indicated for young and active patients, although current published evidence shows no benefit, and, in particular, there is no good evidence that the presence or absence of a TFCC tear affects the outcome.[24] As soon as the intra-articular fragments and soft tissue injuries have been treated, vertical traction is removed, and the VLP is securely fixed to the distal radius.

Advantages of Wrist Arthroscopy

The authors recognize several advantages of arthroscopic surgery for a DRF. First, during PART, apparently better reduction of the articular surface is initially achieved under fluoroscopy, and reduction is reconfirmed by arthroscopy. In this process, the authors noted a difference between fluoroscopic and arthroscopic reduction and hypothesized that after fluoroscopic reduction, there would be no remaining gap and a step-off of 2 mm or more. Under arthroscopy, however, the authors recognized residual displacement of greater than 2 mm in 88 of 273 wrists

intra-articular fractures (22%), particularly in the coronal plane.

In addition, during arthroscopy, the authors found fracture fragments that were not seen on preoperative radiographs and CT scans. In the 273 wrists with displaced intra-articular fractures, free fracture fragments in 25 wrists (9%) were found. If these fragments were not removed, they might in theory produce wrist pain through impingement, although again there is no evidence for this.

VLP should have maximal mechanical effect when the distal screws are inserted into the subchondral zone of the distal radius. If the plate placement is too distal the screws may protrude into the joint surface. Wrist arthroscopy is able to monitor screw protrusion into the joint.

Finally, investigation of the intra-articular soft tissue situation by wrist arthroscopy may be advantageous. Among a total of the 273 wrists, an SLIL injury was seen in 88 wrists (32%). Of these, a total tear was seen in 5 wrists (2%) and repaired in 4 wrists. A traumatic TFCC tear was seen in 159 wrists (45%). A foveal tear with instability of the ulnar head, which was assessed by intraoperative ballottement test and confirmed by arthroscopy, was repaired primarily in 4 wrists (1.4%).

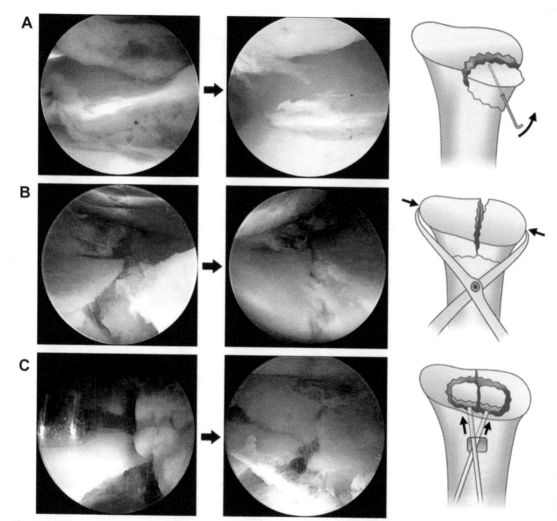

Fig. 5. (*A*) The residual step-off can be reduced with a joy-stick maneuver, (*B*) the gap is reduced by percutaneous tenaculum clamping, and (*C*) a fragment with central depression is reduced by pushing up from the intramedullary canal. Three figures in the *left* column indicate pre-reduction figures, three figures in the *central* column indicate post-reduction figures, and three figures in the *right* column indicate schema of reduction procedure. *Thick arrows* indicate pre- and post-reduction appearance. *Thin arrows* indicate directions of reduction force. (*From* Abe Y. How to perform wrist arthroscopy with volar locking plate fixation for distal radius fracture. MB Orthop 2014;27(1): 79–85; with permission.)

Results

The authors followed 252 wrists treated with PART for a mean of 15 (range: 12–60) months. The mean volar tilt of the distal radius was 6° (range: −10°–16°), the mean radial inclination was 26° (range: 18°–31°), and the mean ulnar variance was 0.1 mm (range: −2–5 mm). The mean extension of the wrist was 69° (range: 50°–85°), and the mean flexion was 63° (range: 35°–79°). The mean pronation of the forearm was 88° (range: 70°–90°), and the mean supination was 89° (range: 75°–95°). The mean grip strength was 90% (range: 31%–133%) of the opposite side. The final results according to the Mayo modified wrist score were 187 excellent (74%), 60 good (24%), 4 fair (2%), and 1 poor. The mean Disabilities of the Arm, Shoulder and Hand (DASH) score at final follow-up was 3.6 (range: 0–33.6).

INTRA-ARTICULAR CORRECTIVE OSTEOTOMY

Failure to reduce the articular surface to less than 2 mm of step-off is considered a cause of posttraumatic osteoarthritis.[25,26] The link with malunion and longer-term symptoms is not supported in many other studies. Several investigators have reported different techniques for intra-articular corrective osteotomy for symptomatic intra-articular malunion, such as arthroscopically assisted osteotomy.[27–29] Even with these techniques, however, it is still difficult to perform an accurate osteotomy through the original fracture line on the articular surface and reduce the malunited fragment to the correct position to reconstruct a smooth joint surface.[30] Arthroscopic procedures require considerable surgical skills. Meanwhile, recent progress in CT imaging and computer technology has enabled simulating an accurate 3-D corrective osteotomy using CT bone models. Furthermore, the development of an intraoperative guiding system that uses a custom-made surgical template makes it possible to perform an operation as simulated preoperatively.[31,32]

This article reports a case of a malunited intra-articular fracture of the distal radius that was treated through an extra-articular approach using a simulated guidance system consisting of an original 3-D computer program and a custom-made surgical guide, which was designed to reproduce a preoperative simulation during the actual

surgery. A 33-year-old man sustained a volar Barton fracture of the right distal radius, which was treated with a forearm plaster cast without reduction. At 7 months after the fracture, the patient complained of wrist pain and restriction of wrist motion. Radiographs showed a 3-mm articular step-off with proximal migration of the ulnovolar fragment of the lunate fossa (**Fig. 6**). To plan corrective surgery for this intra-articular deformity of the distal radius, the authors attempted to simulate a 3-D correction of the deformity using computer models of the bones.[31,32] The correction was planned to be completed by sliding the volar fragment 3 mm distally (**Fig 7**). At operation, the surgical guide was fitted through volar approach, and K-wires (1.2 mm) were passed through a drill sleeve while confirming penetration of the ends through the articular step-off arthroscopically. The osteotomy was accomplished using a chisel along the drill holes. The fragment was

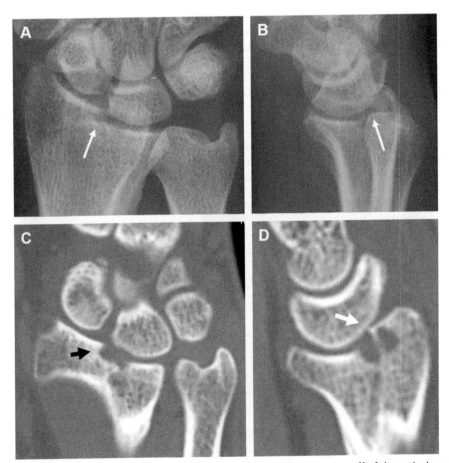

Fig. 6. (*A, B*) Preoperative radiographs and (*C, D*) CT images showing a 3-mm step-off of the articular surface and proximal migration of the ulnar volar fragment. (*A*) Preoperative posteroanterior radiograph. (*B*) Preoperative lateral radiograph. (*C*) Preoperative coronal CT. (*D*) Preoperative sagital CT. *Arrows* indicate a step-off of the articular surface.

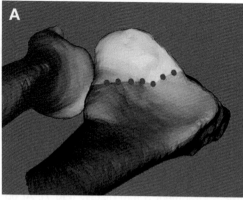
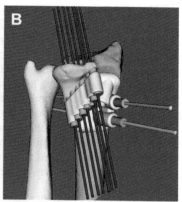

Fig. 7. Computer-assisted planning of an intra-articular osteotomy. (*A*) A planned osteotomy line viewed from the proximal side. (*B*) A customized surgical guide (*white*) equipped with drill holes, through which multiple K-wires (*red*) were set along the osteotomy line. The volar fragment was divided along the step-off and reduced to the level of the original articular surface. To reproduce an intra-articular corrective osteotomy through an extra-articular approach, the authors designed a surgical guide with multiple drill holes using software. Red dotted line indicates the planned osteotomy line in the computer simulation and the customized surgical guide equipped with drill holes through which multiple K-wires were drilled along the osteotomy line.

moved distally by 3 mm and fixed temporarily with 2 K-wires. After the reduction of the articular surface was confirmed arthroscopically and on an image intensifier, the fragment was fixed with a VLP (**Fig 8**).

TRIANGULAR FIBROCARTILAGE COMPLEX AND SCAPHOLUNATE LIGAMENT INTEROSSEOUS LIGAMENT TEARS

Soft tissue injuries associated with a DRF are still challenging diagnostic and therapeutic problems. These injuries cannot be fully detected on preoperative clinical and radiographic evaluations. Moreover, delayed diagnosis may lead to suboptimal outcomes despite healing of the DRF. The TFCC and SL interosseous ligament are 2 major sites of soft tissue tears associated with a DRF. Management of each injury is addressed in this section, and the diagnostic accuracy and reliability of SL gap measurements are described.

Triangular Fibrocartilage Complex Tears

A TFCC tear is the most frequent associated injury and is noted in 39% to 84% of unstable

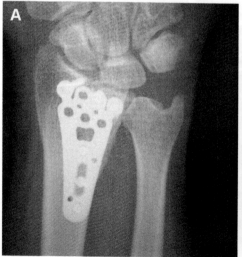
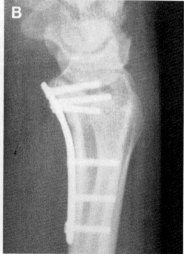

Fig. 8. Postoperative (*A*) anteroposterior and (*B*) lateral radiographs. Anatomic correction and congruity of the radiocarpal joint were obtained. Wrist extension and flexion improved from 30° and 20° preoperatively to 80° and 70°, respectively postoperatively. Grip strength increased from 26 kg to 45 kg, respectively. The patient no longer complained of pain or any functional limitation in activities of daily living.

DRFs.[22,33] The tear locations can be divided into 3 components: triangular fibrocartilage disc, radioulnar ligament (RUL) attachment to the fovea, and the ulnocarpal ligament complex.[34] RUL avulsion at the fovea results in DRUJ instability. Wrist arthroscopy allows a surgeon to diagnose the ligament tear by either indirect or direct techniques. Indirect techniques for the diagnosis include loss of the trampoline effect and the presence of positive hook test,[35,36] whereas direct techniques involve DRUJ arthroscopy to provide direct visualization of the foveal attachment of the ligaments.[34]

DRUJ widening in plain posteroanterior radiographs can predict DRUJ instability accompanying a DRF. Multivariate analyses using a prospective cohort revealed that radial translation of a distal fracture fragment was a significant risk factor for a complete RUL tear.[34,37] Although surgery is probably unnecessary in most cases, several investigators have attempted to repair these ligaments either arthroscopically or at open surgery when there is gross DRUJ instability; they have reported reasonable clinical results.[36,37]

Scapholunate Ligament Tears

SL instability is the most common type of carpal instability; it is found in 32% to 55% of cases based on arthroscopic confirmation.[22,33] In cases of wrist arthroscopy that is unavailable, other imaging modalities have been used for diagnosis. Kwon and Baek[38] evaluated the SL interval by fluoroscopy and concluded that a 2-mm SL gap seemed the best cutoff point for diagnosis of high-grade SL instability based on their arthroscopic findings. Schadel-Hopfner and colleagues[39] reported that preoperative MRI could provide the correct diagnosis of arthroscopically confirmed SL tears in 75% of cases. It seems important to understand the natural course of untreated SL tears. Tang and colleagues[40] identified 20 patients among 424 consecutive patients with DRFs treated nonsurgically who had evidence of radiographic SL dissociation (3.5 ± 0.5 mm).

At 1 year after injury, 18 of 20 patients had fair or poor wrist function by the modified Green and O'Brien scoring system; 8 patients underwent surgery to stabilize the joint. A prospective long-term cohort study investigated the clinical outcomes of patients with arthroscopically confirmed SL tears.[41] No major differences were found in subjective and objective outcomes between complete tears (grade III) and no or partial SL tears (grades I-II); none of the patients developed static SL dissociation or SL advanced wrist collapse, suggesting that grades I-III SL tears can be managed nonsurgically. Although these studies were small and lacked power analyses, the authors summarized that Geissler grades 1 to 3 injuries can be treated nonsurgically. When an SL tear shows SL dissociation (grade IV) together with normal configuration on radiographs of the contralateral wrist, prompt surgical intervention for SL stabilization is recommended.

Diagnostic Accuracy and Reliability of Scapholunate Ligament Gap Measurements

Little is known about the reliability and accuracy of the existing measurement methods of the SL gaps.[42,43] The authors evaluated correlation between arthroscopic and radiographic assessments of SL articulation in 71 consecutive patients who underwent VLP fixation after DRFs. SL instability of all wrists was graded with classification by Geissler and colleagues arthroscopically. Two independent examiners measured the SL intervals at 3 locations (proximal, center, and distal) of the joint on the preoperative posteroanterior wrist radiographs. The radiographic distances were compared between patients with and without SL instability (grades I-III vs grade IV).

The measurements at the center of the joint space differed significantly between the patients with and without SL instability (2.3 mm ± 0.4 mm vs 2.0 mm ± 0.5 mm, respectively; $p<.05$). The area under the receiver operating characteristic curve was 0.74 for identification of SL instability. A cutoff value of 2 mm had 78% sensitivity and 66% specificity. The other measurement methods showed no significant differences between the 2 groups. The intraobserver agreement interclass correlation coefficient value was 0.44 for the central measurement, indicating moderate agreement, 0.11 for the proximal measurement, and 0.19 for the distal measurement. The interobserver interclass correlation coefficient value was 0.11 for the central measurement, indicating slight agreement.

Radiographic measurement at the center of the SL joint space showed higher diagnostic accuracy and reliability than the other measurements, indicating that this is the optimal location for diagnosing associated SL instability but it is still not reliable. Arthroscopically confirmed complete SL ligament tears (grade 4) showed a minimum widening of the central SL joint space of 2 mm, which was lower than the values in previous reports.[44,45]

PROBLEMS RELATED TO THE DISTAL RADIOULNAR JOINT
Extra-articular Malalignment

Extra-articular malalignment of the distal radius can affect DRUJ kinematics, stability, and joint loading. In vivo kinematic studies of the DRUJ have found that contact area of the DRUJ decreased significantly compared with the contralateral uninjured wrist in the malunited distal radius with dorsal angulation.[46,47] Several biomechanical studies investigated effect of extra-articular DRF malalignment on DRUJ stability. Significant DRUJ instability was found after 3 mm of radial shortening, 10° of dorsal and volar angulation, or 2 mm of radial translation.[48–50]

Associated Triangular Fibrocartilage Complex Ligament Tears

The primary stabilizers of the DRUJ are the RULs, that is, the deep portion of the TFCC attaching to the ulnar fovea; complete rupture of the ligaments may contribute to DRUJ instability. The incidence of TFCC injury is correlated with intra-articular involvement and severity of fracture displacement.[51] A long-term prospective cohort study revealed that the natural course of untreated peripheral TFCC tears in distal radial fractures did not provide significant adverse subjective outcomes.[24] Early recognition and treatment of DRUJ instability, however, may lead to better clinical results rather than attempting to manage chronic instability.[52,53] Although accurate diagnosis of RUL tears is difficult, clinical manual stress testing when conducted comparing to the contralateral side provides a practical screening test to differentiate DRUJ instability. A biomechanical study investigated the reliability of the DRUJ ballottement test using cadaver specimens and demonstrated that the ballottement test with a technique of holding the carpal bones to the radius is relatively accurate and reliable for detecting unstable joints.[54]

Intra-articular Malunion of Distal Radioulnar Joint

Intra-articular involvement to the DRUJ occurs in 55% to 65% of displaced DRFs.[55,56] The most frequent fracture line extending into the DRUJ is associated with the dorsoulnar corner fragment of the distal radius; it is best seen on oblique pronated radiographic views. Coronal plane fractures entering the sigmoid notch are more difficult to identify on radiographs. Rozental and colleagues[55] reported that CT scanning revealed fracture extension into the sigmoid notch in 65% of cases, whereas this was only evident in 35% of radiographs. Nakanishi and colleagues[56] analyzed fracture patterns and the magnitude of displacement in the DRUJ by 3D-CT and reported that 28% of the wrists had multiple sigmoid notch fragments (**Fig 9**).

Although previous studies have addressed the issue of intra-articular malunion involving the radiocarpal joint,[57,58] less attention has been paid to the residual gap and step at the DRUJ. It is unclear how intra-articular malunion of the DRUJ would affect functional outcomes. When the displaced fragment is left untreated, residual joint instability or incongruity may lead to degenerative arthritis of the DRUJ, resulting in symptomatic problems. Further studies are needed to clarify how residual malunion at the sigmoid notch would affect functional outcomes.

Functional Outcomes of Intra-articular Fractures Involving The Distal Radioulnar Joint

The authors conducted a prospective cohort study in 58 consecutive patients with Association for Osteosynthesis type C3 DRF treated using volar plating. All patients underwent CT scanning of the injured extremity after manual reduction of the fracture. Axial CT images of the 58 patients were reviewed for the presence, location, and magnitude of fracture displacement involving the DRUJ. There were 31 patients with fracture lines extending into the DRUJ and 27 patients without extension into the DRUJ. The ages of the patients with fractures into the DRUJ (62 ± 12 years old) was significantly higher ($p<.05$) than in patients without (52 ± 20 years old). Of the 31 patients with DRUJ involved fractures, 11 patients had minimally displaced fractures in the DRUJ, 16 had 1 displaced sigmoid notch fracture fragment and 4 had 2 displaced fragments (**Fig 10**); 17 fractures had a step-off or gap greater than or equal to 2 mm and 14 fractures less than 2 mm.

After plate fixation, patients were followed-up for 12 months to 36 months to evaluate postsurgical functional outcomes. The objective outcomes included the ratio of range of injured wrist movement (percent flexion and percent extension) and forearm motion (percent pronation and percent supination) over the nonaffected side, and the ratio of grip strength of the affected hand. DASH scores were derived as a patient-rated measure.

Postoperative percent ranges of wrist and forearm motion in 31 patients were postoperative mean percent ranges of flexion, extension, supination and pronation were 77, 83, 95 and 95, respectively. The percent grip strength was a mean of

Type 0
no fracture in DRUJ

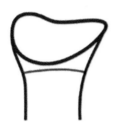

Type 1a
transverse fracture

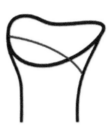

Type 1b
proximal fragment fracture

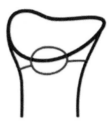

Type 2
longitudinal fracture

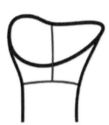

Type 3a
longitudinal fracture with
proximal comminution

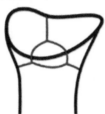

Type 3b
dorsal comminuted fracture

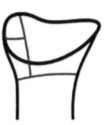

Fig. 9. Type 1a (n = 7) was a transverse fracture in the DRUJ in which fracture lines were not crossing the distal margin of the sigmoid notch. Type 1b (n = 3) was a proximal fragment fracture in which there was a free fragment at the proximal edge of the DRUJ. Type 2 (n = 30), the most common longitudinal fracture, had fracture lines extending into the distal margin of the sigmoid notch. Type 3 has multiple fracture fragments. Type 3a (n = 15) had comminuted fragments at the proximal margin of the DRUJ. Type 3b (n = 5) had comminuted fragments at the dorsal margin of the sigmoid notch. (*From* Nakanishi Y, Omokawa S, Shimizu T, et al. Intra-articular distal radius fractures involving the distal radioulnar joint (DRUJ): three dimensional computed tomography-based classification. J Orthop Sci 2013;18(5): 790; with permission.)

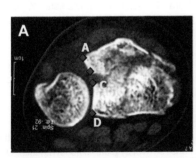

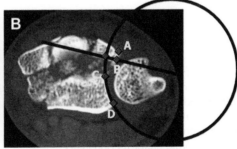

Fig. 10. Gap and step displacement was measured by arc method using a template to trace a circle matching the curvature of the broadest remaining distal radial articular surface. (*A*) The location of fractures at the DRUJ was defined as fraction of width of dorsal fragment (AB) to that of the sigmoid notch (AB + CD) in axial CT image. (*B*) Point A and B indicates each margin of the articular surface of dorsal sigmoid notch fragment, and point C and D indicates that of palmer sigmoid notch fragment. Gap and step were measured as follows: 2 points (B and C) were marked at the fracture margin of the 2 fragments between which displacement was measured. A line was drawn through the geometric center of circle, passing through the margin of the most displaced fragment (point B). The intersection of the line with the arc of the circle was noted as point E. Step displacement was the component of displacement measured along a line between points B and E. Gap displacement was the component of displacement measured between points E and C.

Table 1
Outcomes in patients with distal radioulnar joint incongruity larger or smaller than 2 mm

Evaluation[b]	Displacement at the Sigmoid Notch[a]		
	<2 mm	≥2 mm	P value
Flexion	82 ± 16	70 ± 18	.07
Extension	90 ± 13	75 ± 16	.02[c]
Supination	97 ± 5	92 ± 10	.08
Pronation	94 ± 7	96 ± 8	.50
Grip strength	73 ± 15	77 ± 19	.54
DASH	16 ± 14	17 ± 21	.79

[a] DRUJ incongruity was judged from intra-articular displacement (gap with step) at the sigmoid notch.
[b] Expressed as percentage of the normal except the DASH values.
[c] Statistically significant.

75%; the DASH score was a mean of 17. Statistical analysis showed that only loss of wrist extension was significantly greater in patients with a gap or step larger than 2 mm (**Table 1**).

The current analysis of the data in the 58 patients showed that intra-articular involvement at the sigmoid notch occurred in the elderly. Displacement of an intra-articular fragment of the DRFs greater than or equal to 2 mm was associated with limitation of wrist extension at 1 to 3 years follow-up.

This review was largely based on studies from the authors' teams in Nara and Osaka, Japan and West-Japan, including review of other important literature. Readers' attention is directed to additional recent clinical and basic studies from other Asian groups on the subject of the DRFs.[59–72]

SUMMARY

The watershed line corresponds to the distal margin of the pronator fossa in the radial aspect of the volar radius and to a hypothetical line between the distal and proximal lines in the ulnar aspect. The radial and ulnar bony prominences on the volar radius are key structures for accurate plate placement to avoid flexor tendon injury.

The authors found central depression fragments in 6% of the patients with intra-articular DRF using 3-D CT images, and the depression tends to occur with volar rim fragments in severely comminuted fractures. Radiographic measurement at the center of the SL joint space showed higher diagnostic accuracy and reliability than the other measurements, indicating that this is the optimal location for diagnosing associated SL instability.

Arthroscopically confirmed complete SL ligament tears produced a minimum of 2 mm of SL joint space widening, which was lower than the values in reports from other surgeons. Arthroscopically, the authors found that 22% of the DRFs had residual displacement of greater than 2 mm after fluoroscopically guided surgical reduction and that 9% of these cases had free intra-articular fracture fragments.

ACKNOWLEDGMENTS

The authors thank Tsuyoshi Murase, MD, PhD, at the Department of Orthopedic Surgery, Osaka University Graduate School of Medicine, and Hiroshi Ono, MD, PhD, Ryotaro Fujitani, MD, PhD, and Yasuhito Tanaka, MD, PhD, at the Department of Orthopedic Surgery, Nara Medical University for contributions to this study.

REFERENCES

1. Harness NG, Jupiter JB, Orbay JL, et al. Loss of fixation of the volar lunate facet fragment in fractures of the distal part of the radius. J Bone Joint Surg Am 2004;86A:1900–8.
2. Orbay JL. Volar plate fixation of distal radius fractures. Hand Clin 2005;21:347–54.
3. Imatani J, Akita K, Yamaguchi K, et al. An anatomical study of the watershed line on the volar, distal aspect of the radius: implications for plate placement and avoidance of tendon ruptures. J Hand Surg Am 2012;37:1550–4.
4. Shimizu H, Imatani J, Akita K, et al. Positional relationship between the distal radius and the flexor tendons. J Jpn Socie Surg Hand 2010;27:587–9 [in Japanese].
5. Oura K, Oka K, Kawanishi Y, et al. Volar morphology of the distal radius in axial planes: a quantitative analysis. J Orthop Res 2015;33(4):496–503.
6. Yoneda H, Iwatsuki K, Hara T, et al. Interindividual anatomical variations affect the plate-to-bone fit during osteosynthesis of distal radius fractures. J Orthop Res 2016;34:953–60.
7. Pichler W, Clement H, Hausleitner L, et al. Various circular arc of the distal volar radius and the implications on volar plate osteosynthesis. Orthopedics 2008;31:1–4.
8. Melone CP Jr. Distal radius fractures: patterns of articular fragmentation. Orthop Clin North Am 1993;24:239–53.
9. Trumble TE, Culp RW, Hanel DP, et al. Intra-articular fractures of the distal aspect of the radius. Instr Course Lect 1999;48:465–80.
10. Medoff RJ. Essential radiographic evaluation for distal radius fractures. Hand Clin 2005;21:279–88.

11. Tanabe K, Nakajima T, Sogo E, et al. Intra-articular fractures of the distal radius evaluated by computed tomography. J Hand Surg Am 2011;36:1798–803.

12. Harness NG, Ring D, Zurakowski D, et al. The influence of three-dimensional computed tomography reconstructions on the characterization and treatment of distal radius fractures. J Bone Joint Surg 2006;88A:1315–23.

13. Cole RJ, Bindra RR, Evanoff BA, et al. Radiographic evaluation of osseous displacement following intra-articular fractures of the distal radius: reliability of plain radiography versus computed tomography. J Hand Surg Am 1997;22:792–800.

14. Wagner WF Jr, Tencer AF, Kiser P, et al. Effects of intra-articular distal radius depression on wrist joint contact characteristics. J Hand Surg Am 1996;21:554–60.

15. Doi K, Hattori Y, Otsuka K, et al. Intra-articular fractures of the distal aspect of the radius: arthroscopically assisted reduction compared with open reduction and internal fixation. J Bone Joint Surg 1999;81A:1093–110.

16. Yamazaki H, Uchiyama S, Komatsu M, et al. Arthroscopic assistance does not improve the functional or radiographic outcome of unstable intra-articular distal radial fractures treated with a volar locking plate: a randomised controlled trial. Bone Joint J 2015;97B:957–62.

17. Ruch DS, Vallee J, Poehling GG, et al. Arthroscopic reduction versus fluoroscopic reduction in the management of intra-articular distal radius fractures. Arthroscopy 2004;20:225–30.

18. Abe Y, Tsubone T, Tominaga Y. Plate presetting arthroscopic reduction technique for the distal radius fractures. Tech Hand Up Extrem Surg 2008;12:136–43.

19. Abe Y, Yoshida K, Tominaga Y. Less invasive surgery with wrist arthroscopy for distal radius fracture. J Orthop Sci 2013;18:398–404.

20. Abe Y, Doi K, Hattori Y, et al. A benefit of the volar approach for wrist arthroscopy. Arthroscopy 2003;19:440–5.

21. Abe Y, Doi K, Hattori Y, et al. Arthroscopic assessment of the volar region of the scapholunate interosseous ligament through a volar portal. J Hand Surg Am 2003;28:69–73.

22. Geissler WB, Freeland AE, Savoie FH, et al. Intracarpal soft-tissue lesions associated with an intra-articular fracture of the distal end of the radius. J Bone Joint Surg 1996;78A:357–65.

23. Abe Y, Tominaga Y, Yoshida K. Various patterns of traumatic triangular fibrocartilage complex tear. Hand Surg 2012;17:191–8.

24. Mrkonjic A, Geijer M, Lindau T, et al. The natural course of traumatic triangular fibrocartilage complex tears in distal radial fractures: a 13-15 year follow-up of arthroscopically diagnosed but untreated injuries. J Hand Surg Am 2012;37:1555–60.

25. Trumble TE, Schmitt SR, Vedder NB. Factors affecting functional outcome of displaced intra-articular distal radius fractures. J Hand Surg Am 1994;19:325–40.

26. Bradway JK, Amadio PC, Cooney WP. Open reduction and internal fixation of displaced, comminuted intra-articular fractures of the distal end of the radius. J Bone Joint Surg 1989;71A:839–47.

27. Gobel F, Vardakas DG, Riano F, et al. Arthroscopically assisted intra-articular corrective osteotomy of a malunion of the distal radius. Am J Orthop 2004;33:275–7.

28. del Pinal F, Garcia-Bernal FJ, Delgado J, et al. Correction of malunited intra-articular distal radius fractures with an inside-out osteotomy technique. J Hand Surg Am 2006;31:1029–34.

29. Ring D, Prommersberger KJ, Gonzalez del Pino J, et al. Corrective osteotomy for intra-articular malunion of the distal part of the radius. J Bone Joint Surg 2005;87A:1503–9.

30. Marx RG, Axelrod TS. Intraarticular osteotomy of distal radial malunions. Clin Orthop Relat Res 1996;(327):152–7.

31. Murase T, Oka K, Moritomo H, et al. Three-dimensional corrective osteotomy of malunited fractures of the upper extremity with use of a computer simulation system. J Bone Joint Surg 2008;90A:2375–89.

32. Oka K, Moritomo H, Goto A, et al. Corrective osteotomy for malunited intra-articular fracture of the distal radius using a custom-made surgical guide based on three-dimensional computer simulation: case report. J Hand Surg 2008;33A:835–40.

33. Lindau T, Arner M, Hagberg L. Intraarticular lesions in distal fractures of the radius in young adults. A descriptive arthroscopic study in 50 patients. J Hand Surg Br 1997;22:638–43.

34. Nakamura T, Iwamoto T, Matsumura N, et al. Radiographic and arthroscopic assessment of DRUJ instability due to foveal avulsion of the radioulnar ligament in distal radius fractures. J Wrist Surg 2014;3:12–7.

35. Hermansdorfer JD, Kleinman WB. Management of chronic peripheral tears of the triangular fibrocartilage complex. J Hand Surg Am 1991;16:340–6.

36. Ruch DS, Yang CC, Smith BP. Results of acute arthroscopically repaired triangular fibrocartilage complex injuries associated with intra-articular distal radius fractures. Arthroscopy 2003;19:511–6.

37. Fujitani R, Omokawa S, Akahane M, et al. Predictors of distal radioulnar joint instability in distal radius fractures. J Hand Surg Am 2011;36:1919–25.

38. Kwon BC, Baek GH. Fluoroscopic diagnosis of scapholunate interosseous ligament injuries in distal radius fractures. Clin Orthop Relat Res 2008;466:969–76.

39. Schadel-Hopfner M, Iwinska-Zelder J, Bohringer G, et al. MRI or arthroscopy in the diagnosis of

scapholunate ligament tears in fractures of the distal radius? Handchir Mikrochir Plast Chir 2001;33:234–8.

40. Tang JB, Shi D, Gu YQ, et al. Can cast immobilization successfully treat scapholunate dissociation associated with distal radius fractures? J Hand Surg Am 1996;21:583–90.

41. Mrkonjic A, Lindau T, Geijer M, et al. Arthroscopically diagnosed scapholunate ligament injuries associated with distal radial fractures: a 13- to 15-year follow-up. J Hand Surg Am 2015;40:1077–82.

42. Yin Y, Mann FA, Hodge JC, et al. Roentgenographic interpretation of ligamentous instabilities of the wrist: static and dynamic instabilities. In: Gilula LA, Yin Y, editors. Imaging of the wrist and hand. Philadelphia: WB Saunders; 1996. p. 203–24.

43. Cautilli GP, Wehbe MA. Scapholunate distance and cortical ring sign. J Hand Surg Am 1991;16:501–3.

44. Gilula LA, Weeks PM. Post-traumatic ligamentous instabilities of the wrist. Radiology 1978;129:641–51.

45. Mauel J, Moran SL. The diagnosis and treatment of scapholunate instability. Hand Clin 2010;26:129–44.

46. Xing SG, Chen YR, Xie RG, et al. In vivo contact characteristics of distal radioulnar joint with malunited distal radius during wrist motion. J Hand Surg Am 2015;40:2243–8.

47. Crisco JJ, Moore DC, Marai GE, et al. Effects of distal radius malunion on distal radioulnar joint mechanics–an in vivo study. J Orthop Res 2007;25:547–55.

48. Saito T, Nakamura T, Nagura T, et al. The effects of dorsally angulated distal radius fractures on distal radioulnar joint stability: a biomechanical study. J Hand Surg Eur Vol 2013;38:739–45.

49. Nishiwaki M, Welsh M, Gammon B, et al. Volar subluxation of the ulnar head in dorsal translation deformities of distal radius fractures: an in vitro biomechanical study. J Orthop Trauma 2015;29: 295–300.

50. Day CJ, Jang E, Taylor SA, et al. The impact of coronal alignment on distal radioulnar joint stability following distal radius fracture. J Hand Surg Am 2014;39:1264–72.

51. Richards RS, Bennett JD, Roth JH, et al. Arthroscopic diagnosis of intra-articular soft tissue injuries associated with distal radial fractures. J Hand Surg Am 1997;22:772–6.

52. Geissler WB, Fernandez DL, Lamey DM. Distal radioulnar joint injuries associated with fractures of the distal radius. Clin Orthop Relat Res 1996;327: 135–46.

53. May MM, Lawton JN, Blazar PE. Ulnar styloid fractures associated with distal radius fractures: incidence and implications for distal radioulnar joint instability. J Hand Surg Am 2002;27:965–71.

54. Onishi T, Omokawa S, Iida A, et al. Biomechanical study of distal radioulnar joint ballottement test. J Orthop Res 2016. http://dx.doi.org/10.1002/jor. 23355.

55. Rozental TD, Bozentka DJ, Katz MA, et al. Evaluation of the sigmoid notch with computed tomography following intra-articular distal radius fracture. J Hand Surg Am 2001;26:244–51.

56. Nakanishi Y, Omokawa S, Shimizu T, et al. Intra-articular distal radius fractures involving the distal radioulnar joint (DRUJ): three dimensional computed tomography-based classification. J Orthop Sci 2013;18:788–92.

57. Chung KC, Sandra V, Kotsis H, et al. Predictor of functional outcomes after surgical treatment of distal radius fractures. J Hand Surg Am 2007;32:76–83.

58. Karnezis IA, Panagiotopoulos E, Tyllianakis M, et al. Correlation between radiological parameters and patient-rated wrist dysfunction following fractures of the distal radius. Injury 2005;36:1435–9.

59. Yoon JO, You SL, Kim JK. Intra-articular comminution worsens outcomes of distal radial fractures treated by open reduction and palmar locking plate fixation. J Hand Surg Eur Vol 2017;42:260–5.

60. Wang J, Zhang L, Ma J, et al. Is intramedullary nailing better than the use of volar locking plates for fractures of thedistal radius? A meta-analysis of randomized controlled trials. J Hand Surg Eur Vol 2016; 41:543–52.

61. Tanaka H, Hatta T, Sasajima K, et al. Comparative study of treatment for distal radius fractures with two different palmar locking plates. J Hand Surg Eur Vol 2016;41:536–42.

62. Kasapinova K, Kamiloski V. The correlation of initial radiographic characteristics of distal radius fractures and injuries of the triangular fibrocartilage complex. J Hand Surg Eur Vol 2016;41:516–20.

63. Walenkamp MM, Aydin S, Mulders MA, et al. Predictors of unstable distal radius fractures: a systematic review and meta-analysis. J Hand Surg Eur Vol 2016;41:501–15.

64. Gong HS, Cho HE, Kim J, et al. Surgical treatment of acute distal radioulnar joint instability associated with distal radius fractures. J Hand Surg Eur Vol 2015;40:783–9.

65. Bessho Y, Nakamura T, Nagura T, et al. Effect of volar angulation of extra-articular distal radius fractures on distal radioulnar joint stability: a biomechanical study. J Hand Surg Eur Vol 2015;40: 775–82.

66. Yilmaz S, Cankaya D, Karakus D. Ulnar styloid fracture has no impact on the outcome but decreases supination strength after conservative treatment of distal radial fracture. J Hand Surg Eur Vol 2015;40: 872–3.

67. Nishiwaki M, Welsh MF, Gammon B, et al. Effect of volarly angulated distal radius fractures on forearm rotation and distal radioulnar joint kinematics. J Hand Surg Am 2015;40:2236–42.

68. Chen YR, Xie RG, Tang JB. In vivo changes in the lengths of carpal ligaments after mild dorsal

angulation of distalradius fractures. J Hand Surg Eur Vol 2015;40:494–501.

69. Kodama N, Imai S, Matsusue Y. A simple method for choosing treatment of distal radius fractures. J Hand Surg Am 2013;38:1896–905.

70. Ozasa Y, Iba K, Oki G, et al. Nonunion of the ulnar styloid associated with distal radius malunion. J Hand Surg Am 2013;38:526–31.

71. Roh YH, Lee BK, Baek JR, et al. A randomized comparison of volar plate and external fixation for intra-articular distal radius fractures. J Hand Surg Am 2015;40:34–41.

72. Roh YH, Lee BK, Noh JH, et al. Factors delaying recovery after volar plate fixation of distal radius fractures. J Hand Surg Am 2014;39: 1465–70.

Peripheral Nerve Defects
Overviews of Practice in Europe

Bruno Battiston, MD, PhD*, Paolo Titolo, MD, Davide Ciclamini, MD,
Bernardino Panero, MD

KEYWORDS

• Nerve defect • Autografts • Conduits • Allografts • Nerve transfers • End-to-side

KEY POINTS

- Autologous nerve grafts are the current gold standard for most clinical conditions.
- In selected cases, alternative types of reconstructions can be performed to fill the nerve gap. The use of non-nervous autologous tissue–based conduits (biological tubulization) or synthetic ones is a valuable alternative to short nerve autografts.
- Allografts represent another new field of interest.
- When the nerve defect is severe, nonanatomic solutions may be considered, such as nerve transfers or end-to-side repairs.
- The decision making in the treatment of nerve defects is based on the timing of referral (acute or delayed), the level of the injury (proximal or distal), the type of lesion (closed or open, neat or blunt), and the size of any gap.

INTRODUCTION

High-energy injuries are increasing worldwide driven in part by increasing use of technology in many fields: transport, factories, hobbies, and war. These injuries may cause tissue loss. If nerve continuity is lost, the 2 ends must be bridged to offer the possibility of nerve regeneration and functional restoration.[1–5]

The success of the repair depends on the chosen technique but also on the factors influencing nerve regeneration, primarily patient age and associated diseases, level and site of the lesion (distally nerves are more clearly differentiated toward pure motor or sensory nerves whereas proximal injuries generally involve mixed nerves further from their distal target), mechanism of injury, degree of damage to surrounding tissues, length of the defect, and biological factors (neurotrophic, neurotropic, and neurite-promoting factors).[6,7]

POSSIBILITIES OF NERVE DEFECT REPAIR

The studies carried out by Millesi[1] on the use of interfascicular nerve autografts still represent the gold standard for this kind of injury. Nerve grafts bridge the gap, guide regeneration, and protect axons from the surrounding scar tissue. Generally, the sural nerve is used as the donor or, in some cases, other pure sensitive nerves, such as the medial cutaneous nerve of the arm or forearm and the posterior interosseous nerve at the wrist.

Some investigators described, and used for some years, vascularized nerve grafts, which in theory allow for nerve repair or reconstruction even in avascular beds regardless of graft diameter.[8] Even those investigators who initially reported quicker recoveries compared with traditional small avascular grafts, however, no longer use this technique because its advantages do not justify the complexity of the surgery.

Disclosure: The authors have nothing to disclose.
U.O.C Orthopaedics, Traumatology and Hand Surgery, U.O.D. Microsurgery, C.T.O. Hospital, Via Zuretti 29, Turin 10126, Italy
* Corresponding author.
E-mail address: bruno.battiston@virgilio.it

Harvesting of an autograft creates damage in a sound area: skin scar, sensory loss, and the risk of neuroma formation. Hence, several investigators have looked for new techniques, such as tubes or conduits, without the sacrifice of normal nerves. The tubulization principle represents a biological approach to a nerve injury, in which the role of the surgeon is limited and special emphasis is given to the role of intrinsic healing capacities of the nerve tissue itself inside a guide. Especially in mixed nerves, the regenerating axons are theoretically free to orientate inside a conduit to reach the correct final target.

Although the first tubulization attempts were made using biological material (bone and blood vessels), the idea to use nonbiological materials to bridge a nerve gap came about more recently. Several reports on the use of nonbiological materials (eg, inert metals, permeable cellulose esters, gelatin tubes, rubber, and plastics) for tubulization were published during the twentieth century.[9] In 1955, Garrity[10] reported on the unsuccessful use of polyethylene, polyvinyl, and rubber in 3 patients with very long nerve defects. More recently, Dahlin and Lundborg demonstrated that, in short gaps (less than 5 mm), the use of silicone tubes can lead to successful nerve regeneration.[11] A major concern with the clinical use of nonabsorbable synthetic material in humans is the occurrence of complications due to local fibrosis, induced by the implanted material, and nerve compression.[12] As an alternative to nonabsorbable tubes, bioabsorbable tubes have been tested both experimentally and in clinical practice. In particular, the clinical use of polyglycolic acid conduits has been shown effective for restoring nerve defects.[13,14] Future clinical trials need to demonstrate which of the more recently devised biodegradable materials (for example, chitosan) can be valid alternatives to polyglycolic acid for fashioning conduits for human nerve repair.[15]

Transition to patients of artificial synthetic nerve conduits, however, is still limited despite a large body of preclinical research. On the contrary, the use of non-nervous autologous tissue as grafting material (biological tubulization) received high interest from many researchers and has seen a significant spread into clinics, in selected clinical conditions. This approach is less expensive and avoids complications due to any possible external body inflammatory reaction. Many experimental researches have changed vein grafts with good results,[16] leading to clinical applications.[17] Tissue engineering studies have shown that multiple-component conduits lead to better outcomes in comparison with single-component conduits. In particular, they allow for grafting of longer nerve gaps.

Veins filled with fresh skeletal muscle were first reported in 1993.[18] This biological tissue–engineered tubulization combines 2 elements that have individual limitations. The vein guides regeneration and the muscle prevents vein collapse. Furthermore, the muscle provides an adequate adhesion base for the advancing sprouts by means of neurite-promoting factors present in its basal lamina (laminin and fibronectin), mimicking Schwann cell adhesion. This technique has been applied in several cases since 1993 with good functional results for both sensory and mixed nerves up to 5 cm.[19] These results seem superior to those reported with other kinds of artificial or biological conduits. The conduits come at minimal cost and are prepared according to reconstructive needs after consideration of nerve size and length defect (**Fig. 1**). Recently, more patients have been reviewed who have been treated with the conduits with a range of indications.[20] Especially in emergencies, the use of these biological conduits may avoid the sacrifice of autografts, which could be used for a delayed repair if necessary. Two concepts have guided the development of this technology:

1. The attempt to manipulate different tissues to fashion conduits that mimic some important features of the nerve environment
2. The attempt to enrich hollow biological tubes with elements (laminin and fibronectin) that are considered essential for promoting nerve fiber regeneration and that are generally missing in non-nervous grafts

Some investigators have proposed different tissues, such as human amniotic membrane hollow conduits with autologous skeletal muscle fragments.[21] They used this technique for nerve gaps up to 5 cm with good sensory and motor recovery. Another promising tubulization strategy is use of tissue-engineered tubes made of components of the extracellular matrix, such as collagen.[22] Other types of bioengineered conduits have been experimentally tested but they have not been tried with patients so far. These are based on the enrichment of tubes with laboratory-based elements, such as nerve growth factor,[23] glial growth factor[24] and denatured muscle.[25] Schwann cells used to enrich a hollow conduit[26] seem to hold the most promise because of their central role played in nerve restoration. The first clinical application was recently published where Schwann cells were combined with sural nerve grafts to repair a large sciatic nerve defect after a traumatic nerve injury.[27]

The use of nerve allografts could solve some problems. They have the same structure as a peripheral nerve, so give better adhesion and

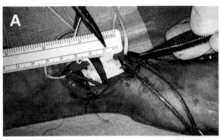
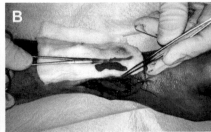
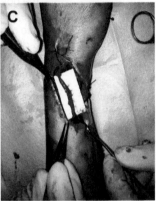

Fig. 1. (*A*) Lesion of the sensory branch of the radial nerve at the wrist with 3-cm defect. (*B*) A piece of muscle is ready to be inserted inside a vein to prepare a muscle-in-vein bioengineered conduit. (*C*) Final reconstruction of the gap without the sacrifice of another sensory nerve autograft.

support to the regenerating axons. The first investigators describing the use of immunogenic grafts needing immunosuppression had poor results.[28] More recently, nonimmunogenic allografts have been developed and used; some initial reports seem encouraging.[29,30] These allografts may be used in gaps up to 7 cm in length as an alternative source of tissue to bolster the diameter of a cable graft and for the management of neuromas in unreconstructable injuries. The neurotropic effect of these grafts may lead to better results compared with empty conduits.[31]

When a nerve lesion with a large gap cannot be repaired by means of an anatomic reconstruction, other systems of functional reinnervation, such as nerve transfers or end-to-side coaptations, may be used. The good clinical experiences of nerve transfers, also called neurotizations, have led to numerous descriptions of nerve transfers. Some investigators have published articles comparing nerve transfers with standard repairs using nerve grafts presenting similar results.[32] The list of possible nerve transfers is long and easily accessible from the literature. On the contrary, even if end-to-side sutures experimentally may represent a new and interesting concept for nerve healing,[33,34] the clinical reports are mixed.[35,36] In the fingers they may represent an alternative to intercalary palmar digital nerve grafts. Currently their

use is limited to cases without other reconstruction options.

CLINICAL APPLICATIONS

Decisions to reconstruct a nerve gap are different in an acute or delayed setting.

Acute Open Injuries

If there is a nerve defect that cannot be apposed with surgical tricks, such as mobilizing the nerve stumps, flexing a joint, or transposing the nerve, the gap needs to be reconstructed. In cases of neat lesions this may be done by means of nerve autografts. Biological or synthetic conduits may be used for short gaps (2–5 cm). If the nerve can be repaired with good surrounding soft tissues, the reconstruction is based on immediate nerve grafting or use of a conduit. If adequate soft tissue coverage is impossible or there is a risk of infection or a need for further débridement, the repair should be delayed. Even in those cases, however, the use of a biological tissue–engineered conduit in an emergency may restore the continuity of the nerve, avoiding secondary nerve graft if function gradually reappears without complications. Even if secondary reconstruction is subsequently required, the secondary surgery may be facilitated by the initial restoration of nerve continuity.[20]

Delayed Repairs

In delayed repairs, the surgeon is usually faced with a scarred bed. After isolation of the nerve lesion, there are typically 2 options: an in-continuity lesion without function needing neuroma resection and reconstruction, or an established nerve gap.

For a nerve-in-continuity, the main problem is to assess the nerve function through electrical stimulation or evoked potentials. If there is no function, the neuroma-in-continuity is resected back to healthy fascicles and the gap reconstructed.

In cases of an established nerve defect, understanding of nerve anatomy (epineurial vessels and internal fascicles orientation, especially if emphasized with methylene blue) may be sufficient to orientate the reconstruction with autografts. Some surgeons describe techniques of identifying the intact fibers and they also try to differentiate motor from sensory fascicles using histology. This approach lengthens surgery, however, and has not shown better results in published clinical series. For short gaps (3–5 cm), engineered conduits or even allografts may represent a good solution because there is theoretic spontaneous orientation of the regenerating axons, which is important, especially in mixed nerves. When surgeons find a very large nerve defect or badly scarred tissues in a proximal lesion with poor prognosis with an anatomic reconstruction, a good alternative may be a distal nerve transfer.[37] Some surgeons preferentially choose a nerve transfer in the reconstruction of some selected nerve lesions.[38,39] Treatment of nerve defects in brachial plexus is not discussed in this review. There seems to be much greater incidence of brachial plexus injuries in Asian regions, although obstetric brachial plexus palsy has similar incidence in Europe with other regions and are often reported.[40–43]

SUMMARY OF METHODS AND DECISION MAKING

To summarize, the choice of reconstruction with autografts or with other is based on the length of the gap, level, and type of injury:

- In multiple trauma patients, the damage control protocol is the rule and the nerve treatment is delayed, waiting for stabilization of a patient.
- In a suitable open wound with a nerve defect, the suggested strategy is nerve grafting or even nerve tubulization depending on the gap length: with loss of nervous tissue greater than 4 cm to 5 cm, autografts are preferred. The nerve repair comes after the treatment of other injuries, if present, for example, bone, tendons, and arteries.
- In extensive open lesions with possible immediate skin coverage (local flap or skin mobilization) again after débridement and treatment of the bone, tendon, and arterial lesions, the nerve defect may be treated immediately and continuity may be restored with a conduit up to 4 cm. Otherwise, nerve autografts represent the gold standard reconstruction.
- In extensive open injuries with difficult soft tissue reconstruction, surgeons should consider 3 different solutions:
  - Coverage with flaps and immediate reconstruction through nerve autografts. This presents some risks, for example, loss of the flap and bad healing with local scar formation compromising the nerve reconstruction.
  - Coverage with flaps and immediate nerve reconstruction by means of conduits. This may be the definitive treatment. In cases of poor nerve recovery, a delayed nerve reconstruction with nerve autografts after 3 months to 6 months can be performed.
  - Soft tissue repair followed by secondary nerve reconstruction through grafts or conduits or even nerve transfers

The decision making can be difficult. Where possible, the aim is safe immediate nerve reconstruction, avoiding the marked scar tissue through good soft tissue coverage. When in doubt, secondary nerve reconstruction is safer. The use of conduits is a choice that leaves open the option of secondary nerve grafting.

In delayed repair of nerve defects, nerve autografts represent the best solution, especially in complex problems, such as brachial plexus injuries. Recent articles, however, have shown that in gaps up to 4 cm to 7 cm, conduits or allografts represent a good option. This approach may progress further with new and interesting research applications. Nonanatomic reconstructions (ie, nerve transfers) are becoming popular especially for very proximal lesions with long distance from the target organ.

REFERENCES

1. Millesi H. Interfascicular nerve grafting. Orthop Clin North Am 1970;2:419–35.
2. Grant GA, Goodkin R, Kliot M. Evaluation and surgical management of peripheral nerve problems. Neurosurgery 1999;44:825–39.
3. Naff NJ, Ecklund JM. History of peripheral nerve surgery techniques. Neurosurg Clin N Am 2001;12:197–209.

4. Campbell WW. Evaluation and management of peripheral nerve injury. Clin Neurophysiol 2008;119: 1951–65.

5. Roganovic Z, Petkovic S. Missile severances of the radial nerve. Results of 131 repairs. Acta Neurochir (Wien) 2004;146:1185–92.

6. Ruijs ACJ, Jaquet JB, Kalmijn S, et al. Median and ulnar nerve injuries: a meta-analysis of predictors of motor and sensory recovery after modern microsurgical nerve repair. Plast Reconstr Surg 2005; 116:484–94.

7. Lundborg G, Dahlin L, Danielsen N, et al. Trophism, tropism and specificity in nerve regeneration. J Reconstr Microsurg 1994;5:345–54.

8. Taylor GI, Ham FJ. The free vascularized nerve graft. A further experimental and clinical application of microvascular techniques. Plast Reconstr Surg 1976;57:413–26.

9. Fields RD, Le Beau JM, Longo F, et al. Nerve regeneration through artificial tubular implants. Prog Neurobiol 1989;33:87–134.

10. Garrity RW. The use of plastic and rubber tubing in the management of irreparable nerve injuries. Surg Forum 1955;6:517–20.

11. Dahlin LB, Lundborg G. Use of tubes in peripheral nerve repair. Neurosurg Clin N Am 2001;12:341–52.

12. Merle M, Dellon AL, Campbell JN, et al. Complications from silicone polymer intubulation of nerves. Microsurgery 1989;10:130–3.

13. Mackinnon SE, Dellon AL. Clinical nerve reconstruction with a bioabsorbable polyglycolic acid tube. Plast Reconstr Surg 1990;85:419–24.

14. LaRosa G, Battiston BA, Sard M, et al. Digital nerve reconstruction with the bioasorbable neurotube. Riv Italiana Chir Plast 2003;35:125–8.

15. Fregnan F, Ciglieri E, Tos P, et al. Chitosan cross-linked flat scaffolds for peripheral nerve regeneration. Biomed Mater 2016;11:045010.

16. Risitano G, Cavallaro G, Lentini M. Autogenous vein and nerve grafts: a comparative study of nerve regeneration in the rat. J Hand Surg Br 1989;14:102–4.

17. Stahl S, Goldberg JA. The use of vein grafts in upper extremity surgery. Eur J Plast Surg 1999;22:255–9.

18. Brunelli G, Battiston B, Vigasio A, et al. Bridging nerve defects with combined skeletal muscle and vein conduits. Microsurgery 1993;14:247–51.

19. Battiston B, Tos P, Cushway T, et al. Nerve repair by means of vein filled with muscle grafts. I. Clinical results. Microsurgery 2000;20:32–6.

20. Tos P, Battiston B, Ciclamini D, et al. Primary repair of crush nerve injuries by means of biological tubulization with muscle-vein-combined grafts. Microsurgery 2012;32:358–63.

21. Riccio M, Pangrazi PP, Parodi PC, et al. The amnion muscle combined graft (AMCG) conduits: a new alternative in the repair of wide substance loss of peripheral nerves. Microsurgery 2014;34:616–22.

22. Li ST, Archibald SJ, Krarup C, et al. Peripheral nerve repair with collagen conduits. Clin Mater 1992;9: 195–200.

23. Gravvanis AI, Tsoutsos DA, Tagaris GA, et al. Beneficial effect of nerve growth factor-7S on peripheral nerve regeneration through inside-out vein grafts: an experimental study. Microsurgery 2004;24:408–15.

24. Mohanna PN, Young RC, Wiberg M, et al. A composite poly-hydroxybutyrate-glial growth factor conduit for long nerve gap repairs. J Anat 2003;203:553–65.

25. Di Benedetto G, Zura G, Mazzucchelli R, et al. Nerve regeneration through a combined autologous conduit (vein plus acellular muscle grafts). Biomaterials 1998;19:173–81.

26. Rodriguez FJ, Verdu E, Ceballos D, et al. Nerve guides seeded with autologous Schwann cells improve nerve regeneration. Exp Neurol 2000;161: 571–84.

27. Levi AD, Burks SS, Anderson KD, et al. Use of autologous Schwann cells to supplement sciatic nerve repair with a large gap: first in human experience. Cell Transplant 2016;25:1395–403.

28. MacKinnon SE. Nerve allotransplantation following severe tibial nerve injury. Case report. J Neurosurg 1996;84:671–6.

29. Safa B, Buncke G. Autograft substitutes: conduits and processed nerve allografts. Hand Clin 2016; 32:127–40.

30. Zhu S, Liu J, Zheng C, et al. Analysis of human acellular nerve allograft reconstruction of 64 injured nerves in the hand and upper extremity: a 3 year follow-up study. J Tissue Eng Regen Med 2016. [Epub ahead of print].

31. Means KR Jr, Rinker BD, Higgins JP, et al. A multicenter, prospective, randomized, pilot study of outcomes for digital nerve repair in the hand using hollow conduit compared with processed allograft nerve. Hand (N Y) 2016;11:144–51.

32. Baltzer HL, Kircher MF, Spinner RJ, et al. A comparison of outcomes of triceps motor branch-to-axillary nerve transfer or sural nerve interpositional grafting for isolated axillary nerve injury. Plast Reconstr Surg 2016;138:256e–64e.

33. Viterbo F, Trinidade JC, Hoshino K, et al. Latero-terminal neurorraphy without removal of epineural sheath in an experimental study in rats. Rev Paul Med 1992;110:267–75.

34. Papalia I, Geuna S, Tos P, et al. Morphologic and functional study of rat median nerve repair by terminolateral neurorrhaphy of the ulnar nerve. J Reconstr Microsurg 2003;19:257–63.

35. Battiston B, Artiaco S, Conforti LG, et al. End-to-side nerve suture in traumatic injuries of brachial plexus: review of the literature and personal case series. J Hand Surg Eur Vol 2009;34:656–9.

36. Artiaco S, Tos P, Conforti LG, et al. Termino-lateral nerve suture in lesions of the digital nerves: clinical experience and literature review. J Hand Surg Eur Vol 2010;35:109–14.

37. Battiston B, Lanzetta M. Reconstruction of high ulnar nerve lesions by distal double median to ulnar nerve transfer. J Hand Surg Am 1999;24:1185–91.

38. Soldado F, Bertelli JA, Ghizoni MF. High median nerve injury: motor and sensory nerve transfers to restore function. Hand Clin 2016;32:209–17.

39. Mackinnon SE. Donor distal, recipient proximal and other personal perspectives on nerve transfers. Hand Clin 2016;32:141–51.

40. Leblebicioglu G, Ayhan C, Firat T, et al. Recovery of upper extremity function following endoscopically assisted contralateral C7 transfer for obstetrical brachial plexus injury. J Hand Surg Eur Vol 2016; 41:863–74.

41. Gibon E, Romana C, Vialle R, et al. Isolated C5-C6 avulsion in obstetric brachial plexus palsy treated by ipsilateral C7 neurotization to the upper trunk: outcomes at a mean follow-up of 9 years. J Hand Surg Eur Vol 2016;41:185–90.

42. Ghanghurde BA, Mehta R, Ladkat KM, et al. Distal transfers as a primary treatment in obstetric brachial plexus palsy: a series of 20 cases. J Hand Surg Eur Vol 2016;41:875–81.

43. Lam WL, Fufa D, Chang NJ, et al. Management of infraclavicular (Chuang Level IV) brachial plexus injuries: A single surgeon experience with 75 cases. J Hand Surg Eur Vol 2015;40:573–82.

Mobilization of Joints of the Hand with Symphalangism

Goo Hyun Baek, MD, PhD*, Jihyeung Kim, MD, PhD, Jin Woo Park, MD

KEYWORDS

- Symphalangism • Congenital anomaly • Hand • Fingers • Mobile joint

KEY POINTS

- Symphalangism of the hand can be classified into 3 grades, from I to III, based on histology.
- Joints with grade I and early grade II symphalangism can achieve some mobility with surgery and aggressive postoperative rehabilitation.
- The age of the patient is important in considering surgery. The earlier the operation, the better the results.

INTRODUCTION

Symphalangism can be defined as congenital ankylosis of the interphalangeal (IP) joints of the fingers or toes. In the hand, the proximal IP (PIP) joint is the most commonly involved; the distal IP (DIP) joint and thumb IP joint can also be involved. Sometimes, both the PIP and DIP joints are affected in the same finger. The metacarpophalangeal (MP) joint can be involved; however, this condition might be better described as MP ankylosis or MP synostosis to prevent confusion. The affected joints are usually ankylosed in extension. Transverse dorsal skin creases are usually faint or not seen over the skin of the affected joint. A slight decrease of the width or length of the affected finger may be seen.

In 1838, Mercier[1] reported on a 22-year-old man who had only 2 phalanges on each finger; this is considered as the first report on symphalangism. Cushing[2,3] reported on a family who had hereditary ankylosis of PIP joints, and first introduced the term symphalangism. Other terminologies, including phalangeal anarthrosis,[4] orthodactyly,[5] and ankylosing arthropathy,[6] have been proposed, although they are seldom used.

The literature on the incidence of symphalangism is very limited. In his series, Flatt[7] concluded that symphalangism accounted for 0.03% of all congenital anomalies of the upper limb; this was 0.04% in the series by Ogino and colleagues.[8]

Symphalangism was used to describe an autosomal dominant disorder affecting PIP joints of the fingers in the early twentieth century.[2–4,6] Most of these cases are related to the mutations of the NOG or noggin gene.[9–11] However, many investigators have included congenitally stiff DIP and MP joints into reports on symphalangism.[12–16] Thalidomide-induced symphalangism was also reported.[13] The nonhereditary symphalangism often

Financial Disclosure: No commercial or financial conflicts to disclose.
Department of Orthopedic Surgery, Seoul National University College of Medicine, 101 Daehak-no, Jongno-gu, Seoul 03080, Republic of Korea
* Corresponding author.
E-mail address: ghbaek@snu.ac.kr

hand.theclinics.com

seen with symbrachydactyly has been reported sporadically.[14] Most of the authors' patients with symphalangism did not have a family history.

Flatt and Wood[12] classified symphalangism into 3 groups: true symphalangism; symbrachydactylism in which the digits are short and stiff; and symphalangism and syndactylism, which includes Apert syndrome and Poland syndrome. A finger with true symphalangism is usually shorter or more slender than adjacent digits but sometimes of normal length.

There have been several reports on techniques to mobilize fingers with symphalangism.[13,17] In 4 adult patients with true symphalangism, silicone rubber implants were inserted into the PIP joints of middle fingers and 50° of motion was reported

at a follow-up of 2 to 4 years.[17] In a 6-year-old child, a vascularized toe joint transfer to the ring finger PIP joint resulted in a reasonable range of motion (ROM) at 4 years follow-up.[13] However, most procedures to mobilize affected joints have been reported to yield unsatisfactory functional results.[12,15,16] In 2012, Baek and Lee[18] reported a new surgical technique mobilize fingers with symphalangism.[18] Thirty-six joints in 17 children were treated surgically; 30 gained a mean of 47° at a mean follow-up of 30 months.

NATURAL HISTORY

The authors had an opportunity to observe a girl with multiple symphalangism of the bilateral

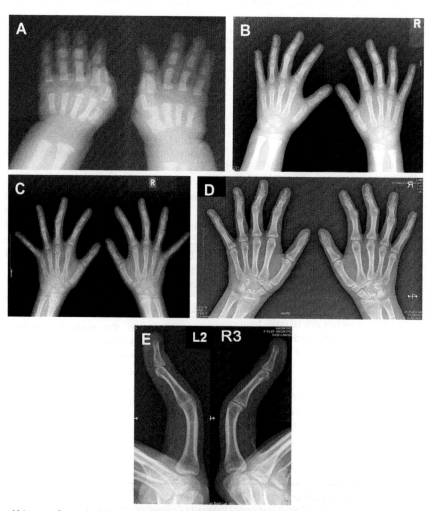

Fig. 1. Natural history of symphalangism. (*A*) Mild joint space narrowing was observed in all the PIP joints except for the right fifth joint. (*B*) Progression of joint space narrowing was observed at age 7 years. (*C*) Joint spaces were barely seen at age 10 years. (*D*) When she was 18 years old, all the epiphyseal plates were closed, and both thumb IP joints, right fourth PIP joint, and left third, fourth, and fifth PIP joints showed bony symphalangism. (*E*) The right third PIP and left second PIP joints showed faint flat joint spaces in simple radiographs although there was no active motion.

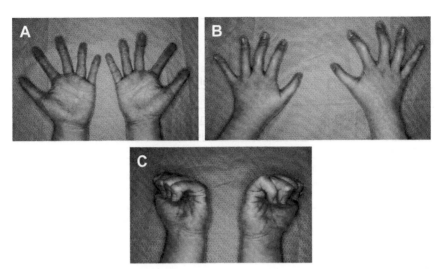

Fig. 2. (*A–C*) Gross appearance and active ROM of the patient. The right fifth finger, which was the only unaffected digit, was slightly longer and wider than affected left fifth finger. Compensatory hyperflexion of the DIP joints was observed in affected fingers.

hands, from 2 months of age till 18 years of age (**Fig. 1**). When the baby visited our clinic at the age of 2 months, there was no active motion at all the PIP joints except for the right fifth joint. Likewise, there was no motion in the thumb IP joints bilaterally. Skin creases over the affected joints were absent or very faint. On simple radiographs, the joint spaces were mildly narrowed in the affected fingers when compared with those of DIP joints (see **Fig. 1**A). When she became 7 years old, the joint space narrowing was more aggravated in the affected joints (see **Fig. 1**B). At the age of 10 year, joint spaces were barely seen in simple radiographs (see **Fig. 1**C). When she became 18 years old, all the epiphyseal plates were closed, and both thumb IP joints, right fourth PIP joint, and left third, fourth, and fifth PIP joints showed bony symphalangism (see **Fig. 1**D). The right second and third PIP and left second PIP joints showed faint joint spaces in simple radiographs, although there was no active motion (see **Fig. 1**E). Her right

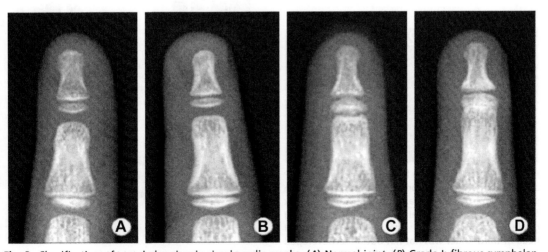

Fig. 3. Classification of symphalangism in simple radiographs. (*A*) Normal joint. (*B*) Grade I: fibrous symphalangism, mild joint space narrowing in DIP joint. (*C*) Grade II: cartilaginous symphalangism, only slit of joint space is observed. (*D*) Grade III: bony symphalangism. (*From* Baek GH, Lee HJ. Classification and surgical treatment of symphalangism in interphalangeal joints of the hand. Clin Orthop Surg 2012;4(1):59; with permission.)

Table 1
Classification of symphalangism

	Grade I (Fibrous Symphalangism)	Grade II (Cartilaginous Symphalangism)	Grade III (Bony Symphalangism)
Volar Skin Crease	Faint or absent	Absent	Absent
Active Motion	Absent	Absent	Absent
Passive Motion	10°–20°	Only jerk of motion	Absent or jerk of motion
Simple radiographs			
Joint space	Mild narrowing	Definite narrowing	Joint space absent
Phalangeal head in Lateral view	Round	Flat	Fused to adjacent bone

Adapted from Baek GH, Lee HJ. Classification and surgical treatment of symphalangism in interphalangeal joints of the hand. Clin Orthop Surg 2012;4(1):60; with permission.

fifth finger, which was the only unaffected digit, was slightly longer and wider than the affected left fifth finger. Compensatory hyperflexion of the DIP joints was observed in affected fingers (**Fig. 2**). None of her family had history of symphalangism.

In the authors' experiences, patients with symphalangism typically present with absent or very faint skin creases over the affected joints. In many young children with symphalangism, simple radiographic findings are deceptive because apparent joint spaces are visible between both ends of 2 adjacent bones, even when there is no movement.[12,18,19] Joint space narrowing will typically become more marked with time until joint spaces are barely visible radiologically. The joints may progress to bony symphalangism by the time of epiphyseal plate closure. In PIP joint symphalangism, compensatory hyperflexion of the DIP joints may be seen.

Classification

As demonstrated in **Figs. 1** and **2**, symphalangism is a progressive condition going from an immobile fibrous joint to a fused joint. It can be classified into 3 grades based on the histology: fibrous; cartilaginous; and bony symphalangism.[18] The radiographic and clinical characteristics of each grade are summarized in **Fig. 3** and **Table 1**.

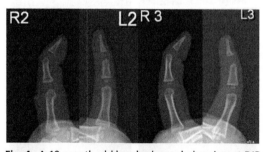

Fig. 4. A 19-month-old boy had symphalangism at DIP and PIP joints of left second and third fingers. The proximal and middle phalangeal heads of the index finger were flat in lateral radiographs, suggesting grade II symphalangism. The middle phalangeal head of third finger was not flat but underdeveloped compared with that of the right side (grade I). However, the proximal phalangeal head was flat (grade II). The index PIP joint space was slightly narrower than that of the third PIP joint.

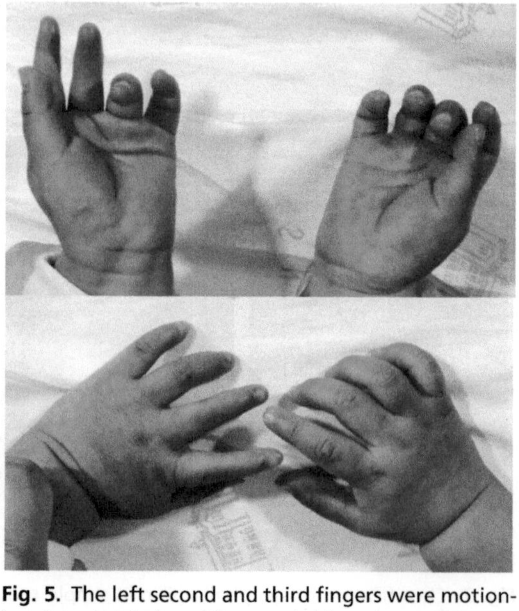

Fig. 5. The left second and third fingers were motionless in extended position, and skin creases were not observed volarly (*top*) and dorsally (*bottom*). The fingers were thinner and slightly shorter than normal side.

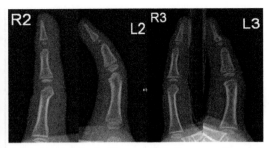

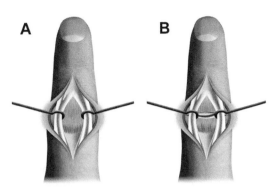

Fig. 6. Two and a half years after the operation, left index PIP joint was fused (second from left) but the third PIP joint (second from right) maintained joint space and congruity.

Fig. 8. (*A, B*) Longitudinal tendon splitting approach.

In grade I, a small amount of passive motion is possible because surrounding soft tissues, including collateral ligaments and joint capsule, are not as stiff as bone. There is a visible joint space radiologically. However, surrounding soft tissues are too tight to allow passive joint movement. There are often faint dorsal skin creases over the affected joint.

In grade II, the fingers are typically virtually ankylosed. There is virtually no passive and no active movement. At operation, a small slit of joint space can sometimes be seen. However, there is typically a solid mass of hyaline cartilage linking the bone ends. Grade II fingers might be further subclassified into early grade II, which have a small joint space, and late grade II, which have no joint space. Sometimes it is not easy to distinguish grade I from early grade II. If there is visible passive motion and faint but distinct skin creases, grade I

is more likely. On simple lateral radiograph of the affected finger, the phalangeal head is round in grade I and flat in grade II (**Fig. 4**). At operation in early grade II symphalangism, there is peripheral cartilaginous fusion of the affected joint but central joint space is visible, although it is narrowed. Fine dissection during surgery may separate both ends of 2 bones smoothly; however, carving of the fused cartilaginous portion sometimes yields incongruity of the joint and subsequent stiffness postoperatively. In late grade II symphalangism there is a complete cartilaginous mass between the adjacent bone ends with no joint space. Careful surgical separation and carving of the cartilaginous mass usually results in little long-term gain with postoperative stiffness.

Surgical outcomes are usually good for grade I joints, mixed for early grade II (see **Figs. 4–7**), and poor for late grades II and III.

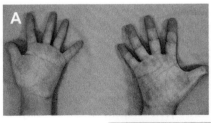

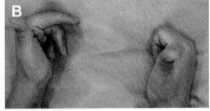

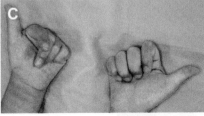

Fig. 7. Both PIP joints were operated on. During the operation, the index PIP joint was confirmed as late grade II, and the third as early grade II. (*A–C*) Four and a half years after the operation, 80° of active flexion was observed at third PIP joint although no active motion was found at the index PIP joint.

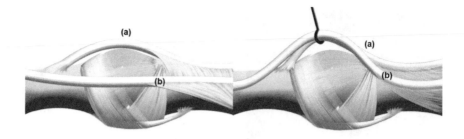

Fig. 9. Retracting lateral band approach without tendon splitting. (a) Central tendon. (b) Lateral band.

Diagnosis

The physical findings are the most important for diagnosis of symphalangism. Skin creases over the affected joint are absent or faint. The affected fingers may sometimes be slightly short and narrow. Active or passive motion is limited or not possible at all, depending on the grade. Bilateral AP and lateral radiographs of all fingers are necessary to show the degree of joint fusion and to compare affected fingers with normal ones. On simple radiographs, the amount of joint space narrowing and the shape of phalangeal head are very helpful for diagnosis and grading. In the authors' experiences, absent flexor or extensor tendons are not seen in true symphalangism. The flexor tendons can usually be palpated during careful examination. Ultrasonography is helpful to evaluate the presence and size of any tendons. MRI scans are usually not helpful because the fingers are too small.

Surgical Indications

In the authors' opinions, surgery is not indicated for symphalangism in symbrachydactyly because the fingers are too small and the extrinsic and intrinsic tendons and muscles are hypoplastic or absent. Surgery is not indicated for symphalangism associated with syndromic syndactyly, such as Apert hand or Poland syndrome, because of the pathologic complexity.

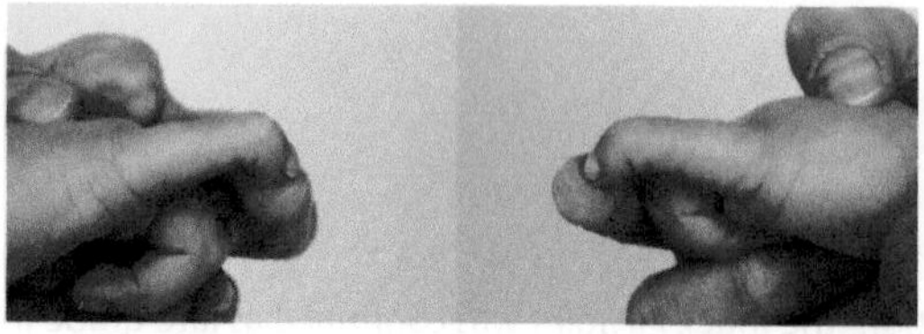

The ideal surgical indications include grade I PIP or DIP joint symphalangism treated between 18 and 24 months of age.[18] When the operation is performed before 18 months of age, it is not easy to handle tiny structures and the postoperative physical therapy is difficult. Grade I or early grade II thumb IP symphalangism may yield good surgical outcome if treated up to 5 years of age.

Lesser indications include grade I PIP or DIP joint symphalangism treated in patients aged 2 to 3 years, early grade II PIP or DIP joint symphalangism treated between 18 and 24 months of age, and grade I or early grade II thumb IP joint symphalangism treated before the age of 7 years.

After 36 months of age, most of the affected joints have progressed from grade I to grade II. However, the rate of progression is slower in thumb IP joints. Thus, the age of the patient is one of the most important factors in considering surgery. Surgical release of the PIP joint only is recommended if both DIP and PIP joints are affected in the same finger. The PIP joint is more important for hand function; simultaneous operations on both joints may cause wound problems or more pain during postoperative physical therapy. Isolated DIP joint symphalangism is not troublesome in most patients. However, surgical treatment is only recommended when the parents of these patients want their young children to have jobs or hobbies that need DIP joint motion, such as playing a musical instrument.

Surgical Technique

Proximal interphalangeal joint

Via a longitudinal dorsal incision centered on the PIP joint (a Z-plasty incision is not necessary), a longitudinal incision is made on the midline of the extensor apparatus. The extensor tendon is carefully separated from underlying joint capsule and collateral ligaments (**Fig. 8**A). Then the dorsal

Fig. 10. Fifteen-month-old boy showed grade I bilateral fifth PIP symphalangism.

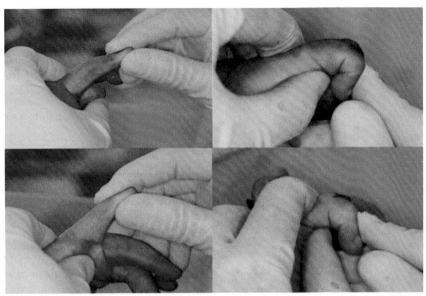

Fig. 11. Both PIP joints were passively flexed 90° intraoperatively. (*From* Baek GH, Lee HJ. Classification and surgical treatment of symphalangism in interphalangeal joints of the hand. Clin Orthop Surg 2012;4(1):61; with permission.)

half of the joint capsule is incised transversely to inspect the inside of the joint (see **Fig. 8**B). In grade I joints, articular cartilages are well separated proximally and distally. In early grade II joints, only a slit of joint space is observed; the peripheral portion of the joint is connected by cartilaginous tissue. The dorsal halves of both the medial and lateral collateral ligaments are divided transversely. For early grade II joints, gentle separation of the peripheral cartilaginous tissue is necessary. In grade I joints, gentle passive flexion always achieves full flexion. On the other hand, more forceful passive flexion is needed in early grade II joints. Passive flexion of the joint may produce a popping sound or sensation. When passive flexion is not enough, the authors believe that release of proximal part of volar plate using small blunt periosteal elevator is

sometimes necessary to improve flexion by loosening the joint. At the end the extensor tendon and skin are repaired.

Alternatively, the lateral band is retracted dorsally by a skin hook after splitting or cutting overlying transverse retinacular ligament (**Fig. 9**). The dorsal capsule and dorsal half of the collateral ligaments are divided.

Thumb interphalangeal joint or finger distal interphalangeal joint

A Y-shaped dorsal incision is made. After retracting the skin, the extensor tendon is dissected from the joint. The dorsal capsule and dorsal halves of bilateral collateral ligaments are divided.

Postoperatively, a simple dressing using Coban (3M, Minneapolis, MN) is applied. From 1 or

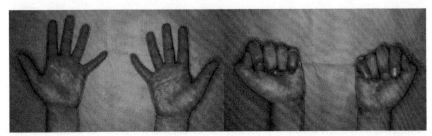

Fig. 12. Three and half years after the operation, right fifth PIP joint showed 90° of active flexion, and left 80°.

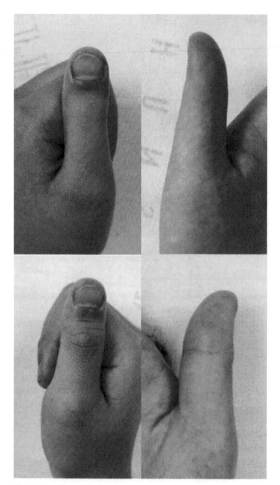

2 days postoperatively, gentle passive ROM exercise is started by hand therapists and parents. At least 4 30-minute sessions of passive ROM exercises a day are recommended. The patients may need brain education to actively flex the joints, probably because the brain motor cortices for affected fingers have not yet been formed. The authors recommend postoperative exercise for a minimum of 6 months.

Outcomes

In the study by Baek and Lee,[18] surgical outcomes were better when patients with symphalangism were operated before the age of 24 months. The initial postoperative active ROM reduced until 2 years postoperatively; thereafter the ROM remained unchanged.[18]

Since 2004, the authors have operated on 63 grade I and II joints; 36 patients have been operated on and followed up for more than 1 year by a single surgeon (GHB). Fifty-two were PIP joints (28 patients; 13 boys and 15 girls), 4 DIP joints (3 patients; 2 boys and one girl), and 7 thumb IP joints (6 patients; 3 boys and 2 girls).

Two patients had family history affecting their fathers. The mean age at operation was 42 (range 15–113) months. Since 2010, most patients have been operated on before the age of 3 years. In 6 of the 63 joints, a complete loss of motion was found in the long term, at an average of 17° (range 0°–45°) flexion. All were grade II PIP joints. The mean gain of active flexion in the remaining 58 joints was 65° (range 0°–100°). The duration of follow-up was a mean of 34 (range 1–12) months.

Fig. 13. A boy who was 6 years and 10 months old had symphalangism of left thumb IP joint (*top pictures*). Left thumb was motionless, smaller than right thumb (*bottom pictures*), and did not show skin creases.

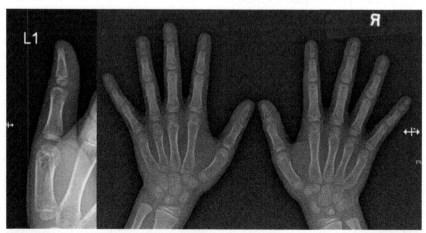

Fig. 14. The joint space of the left thumb IP joint was narrowed, and the proximal phalangeal head was flat in lateral view (*left*), suggesting early grade II symphalangism.

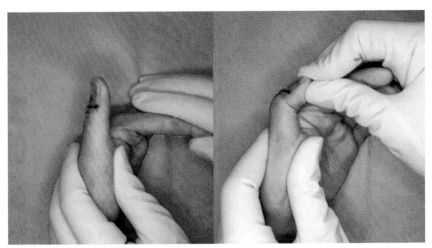

Fig. 15. Passive ROM of 50° was observed intraoperatively.

Proximal interphalangeal joints

Fifty-two PIP joints were treated in 28 patients: index 6, middle 10, ring 7, and little finger 29 (**Figs. 10–12**). Forty joints were grade I and 12 were grade II. In the 12 grade II joints, 6 suffered recurrent ankylosis postoperatively even though intraoperative passive ROMs were more than 50°. Among the 28 operated patients, 15 had multiple joint involvement. In 15 fingers in 6 patients, both PIP and DIP joints were involved.

Thumb interphalangeal joints

The authors treated 7 thumb IP joints in 6 patients: 6 were grade I and 2 were grade II (**Figs. 13–16**). All the joints were mobile postoperatively; their active ROMs ranged from 20° to 60°. Even in the 3 patients who were aged 67, 72, and 94 months at the time of surgery, the postoperative active ROM ranged from 20° to 50°.

Distal interphalangeal joints

The authors treated 4 DIP joints in 3 patients: all were grade I. At follow-up at a mean of 34 (range 15–74) months, all the joints were mobile. Their active ROMs were a mean of 47° (range 30°–60°).

SUMMARY

Based on our experiences, the authors were able to classify symphalangism of the hand into 3 grades and suggest surgical indications. Grade I and early grade II joints can be mobilized with early surgical intervention. Surgical results may vary, but even a 20° gain in motion could be helpful for the child and their parents. Postoperative passive ROM exercises are very important in maintaining mobility of the joints. It is important that the parents understand exercise may cause some pain and that they must be motivated to help their children during the rehabilitation period.

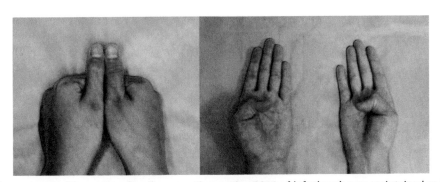

Fig. 16. Three years and 2 months after the operation, active ROM of left thumb was maintained as 50°.

REFERENCES

1. Mercier LA. Absence héréditaire d'une phalange aux doigts et aux orteils. Bull de la Société Anatomique de Paris 1838;13:35–42.
2. Cushing H. Hereditary anchylosis of the proximal phalangeal joints (symphalangism). Proc Natl Acad Sci U S A 1915;1:621–2.
3. Cushing H. Hereditary anchylosis of the proximal phalangeal joints (symphalangism). Genetics 1916; 1:90–106.
4. Drinkwater H. Phalangeal anarthrosis (synostosis, ankylosis) transmitted through fourteen generations. Proc R Soc Med 1917;10(Pathol Sect):60–8.
5. Duncan FN. Orthodactyly. J Hered 1917;8:174–5.
6. Bloom AR. Hereditary multiple ankylosing arthropathy. Radiology 1937;29:166–71.
7. Flatt AE. The care of congenital hand anomalies. St. Louis (MO): Mosby; 1977. p. 146–70.
8. Ogino T, Minami A, Fukuda K, et al. Congenital anomalies of the upper limb among the Japanese in Sapporo. J Hand Surg 1986;11B:364–71.
9. Polymeropoulos MH, Poush J, Rubenstein JR, et al. Localization of the gene (SYM1) for proximal symphalangism to human chromosome 17q21-q22. Genomics 1995;27:225–9.
10. Takahashi T, Takahashi I, Komatsu M, et al. Mutations of the NOG gene in individuals with proximal symphalangism and multiple synostosis syndrome. Clin Genet 2001;60:447–51.
11. Takano K, Ogasawara N, Matsunaga T, et al. A novel nonsense mutation in the NOG gene causes familial NOG-related symphalangism spectrum disorder. Hum Genome Var 2016;3:16023.
12. Flatt AE, Wood VE. Rigid digits or symphalangism. Hand 1975;7:197–214.
13. Shibata M. Symphalangism. In: Gupta A, KAy SPL, Scheker LR, editors. The growing hand. 1st ed. London: Mosby; 2000. p. 289–92.
14. Upton J. Failure of differentiation and overgrowth. In: Mathes SJ, Hentz VR, editors. Plastic surgery. 2nd edition. Philadelphia: WB Saunders; 2006. p. 265–9.
15. Dobyns J. Symphalangism. In: Green DP, Hotchkiss RN, Pederson WC, editors. Green's operative hand surgery. 4th edition. New York: Churchill Livingstone; 1999. p. 470–3.
16. Ogino T. In: Buck-Gramcko D, editor. Congenital malformations of the hand and forearm. 1st edition. London: Churchill Livingstone; 1998. p. 341–4.
17. Palmieri TJ. The use of silicone rubber implant arthroplasty in treatment of true symphalangism. J Hand Surg Am 1980;5:242–4.
18. Baek GH, Lee HJ. Classification and surgical treatment of symphalangism in interphalangeal joints of the hand. Clin Orthop Surg 2012;4:58–65.
19. Takagi R, Kawabata H, Matsui Y. Thumb polydactyly with symphalangism in young children. J Hand Surg Eur 2009;34:800–4.

Common Hand Problems with Different Treatments in Countries in Asia and Europe

Jin Bo Tang, MD[a],*, Grey Giddins, FRCS (Orth), EDHS[b],*,
Shohei Omokawa, MD, PhD[c],
Michel E.H. Boeckstyns, MD, PhD[d], Shian Chao Tay, MD[e],
Thomas Giesen, MD[f]

KEYWORDS

- Fingertip defect • Replantation • Tendon repair • Mallet finger • Carpal ligament injury
- Distal radius fracture • Nerve compression

KEY POINTS

- Distal pulp defects or amputation in the fingertip can be treated with either a flap transfer or dressing changes. Dressing changes can be used even in patients with exposure of the distal phalanx but may take several weeks or over 1 month to 2 months to heal. This is a popular method of treatment in Europe.
- Distal digital tip replantation is performed by some Asian microsurgeons but rarely in Europe. Replacing the amputated tip as a composite graft is common practice in children.
- A peripheral tendon suture is less important and less mandatory when a strong core suture repair is used in flexor tendon repair. Some European surgeons do not use a peripheral suture and still have good outcomes.
- Mallet finger with greater than one-third articular involvement is mostly treated nonoperatively but surgically depending on displacement or joint subluxation, but the degrees of subluxation or fracture displacement, which leads to surgery, vary greatly.
- The indications for use of wrist arthroscopy in assisting surgical reduction and internal fixation of intra-articular distal radius fracture vary greatly. The need of immediate repair of disrupted carpal ligaments at the time of this surgery is neither defined nor agreed.
- All agree that clinical entities, such as thoracic outlet syndrome, complex regional pain syndrome (CRPS), radial tunnel syndrome, pronator syndrome, and radial tunnel syndrome, exist, but their diagnosis is subjective. In making a diagnosis, a second opinion should be sought, and in treating these patients, spontaneous recovery of these conditions in most patients should always be clearly recognized.

INTRODUCTION

Common hand problems are treated differently in different countries. This article attempts to bring together the views of surgeons from different countries on some of the most common hand problems that hand surgeons encounter in daily

The authors have nothing to disclose.
[a] Department of Hand Surgery, The Hand Surgery Research Center, Affiliated Hospital of Nantong University, 20 West Temple Road, Nantong 226001, Jiangsu, China; [b] The Hand to Elbow Clinic, 29a James Street West, Bath BA1 2BT, UK; [c] Department of Hand Surgery, Nara Medical University, Nara, Japan; [d] CFR Hospitals, Hellerup, Denmark; [e] Department of Hand Surgery, Singapore General Hospital, Singapore, Singapore; [f] Plastic Surgery and Hand Surgery Division, University Hospital Zurich, Zurich, Switzerland
* Corresponding author.
E-mail addresses: jinbotang@yahoo.com (J.B.T.); greygiddins@thehandclinic.co.uk (G.G.)

Hand Clin 33 (2017) 561–569
http://dx.doi.org/10.1016/j.hcl.2017.04.010

practice. In practice, the correct treatment of these problems may be the most important and influential to patients. The lead author, JB Tang, formulated several questions, which were sent to 6 senior hand surgeons from 6 countries—3 in Asia and 3 in Europe—for them to give views and comments. Their replies are presented.

DIGITAL SOFT TISSUE REPAIRS

Question: I know Dr Omokawa worked on the anatomy of small vascularized flaps from the hand for digital repairs and also used these flaps in practice. My questions to Dr Omokawa are as follows. Dr Omokawa, do you or (or other Japanese hand surgeons) use these flaps often and what comments do you have on small intrinsic flaps from the hand if your patients have small soft tissue defect; what is your choice—a pedicled flap, a free flap, or something else? Dr Tay, can you tell us the preferred methods in Singapore? I also would like to know the views on fingertip repairs from European colleagues. I know that not performing a flap transfer, leaving the wound in a moist condition with dressing changes, is common in European countries. My impression is that European colleagues treat those tip defects with occlusive dressings, allowing self-regeneration more often than Asian surgeons. Do you use flaps or simply do dressings and let the wound regenerate?

Shohei Omokawa

In Japan, plastic hand surgeons prefer to use intrinsic hand flaps for digital soft tissue defects more frequently than orthopedic hand surgeons. Recent perforator flap reconstruction enables a range of soft tissue coverage in hand surgery.[1]

My indications for flap surgery in digital soft tissue defects are:

1. Skin and soft tissue defects with exposed bone, tendons, or nerve
2. Fingertip injuries with a massive pulp defect

For small soft tissue defects, I use occlusive dressing. Reverse homodigital artery flaps are rarely indicated because 1 of the palmer digital arteries is sacrificed. A pedicled cross-finger, a thenar flap, or a free flap also is rarely used in my practice.

For most cases, I use 1 of 2 homodigital island flaps for reconstruction of soft tissue defects. The first is a neurovascular pedicle volar advancement flap, and the second is dorsal middle phalangeal perforator–based propeller flap with innervation by the dorsal digital nerve branch.[2]

The clinical result from in our unit, however, measured with the pegboard performance test was not satisfactory in patients with flap surgery in the index or middle fingers. Comparison of the test between using the injured finger and the adjacent normal finger revealed that the score of the affected finger was worse than that of the adjacent finger, indicating that digital performance after reconstruction with this flap was still limited despite the patients showing high satisfaction and good sensory recovery. I anticipate that future novel approaches can overcome the limitation of flap surgery to produce cosmetic and functional result equal to those of the adjacent finger.

Shian Chao Tay

For fingertip defects more than 1 cm^2, I prefer a cross-finger flap followed by V-Y plasty. Some surgeons also use a thenar flap. We have had good outcomes with the cross-finger flap, which is a reliable workhorse flap for fingertip resurfacing. Other options for these larger defects include:

1. Homodigital flaps, for example, the spiral flap[3] and the neurovascular island flap[4]
2. Heterodigital flaps, for example, the heterodigital arterialized flap,[5] which does not take the digital nerve and leaves the pulp of the donor finger intact

The heterodigital arterialized flap may be harvested with a dorsal vein to enhance venous return. In situations where the dorsal vein affects flap transfer, the vein can be divided and then reanastomosed after flap transfer.[6]

Thomas Giesen

We use the moist dressing in Allen zone 1. In zone 2 it is more dependent on the experience of the surgeon. Our workhorse flaps for the fingertip are the V-Y and the Segmüller flaps. If the bone is exposed or if the volume missing will result in a square fingertip, we then use normally a local flap.

Michel Ernest H. Boeckstyns

In my country, Denmark, we rely on the ability of spontaneous regeneration of the skin of the pulp and, whenever possible, use conservative treatment with changing of dressings until healing. There are a variety of regimens to achieve this. Pulp regeneration tends to give good results with preserved sensibility and minimal scar problems.

If some phalangeal bone is prominent, I revise it carefully with a rongeur. In patients with a tangential amputation and a larger area of uncovered bone, I use a Moberg flap or a kite flap in the thumb and advancement flaps in the fingers.

Grey Giddins

Mostly we take a minimalist approach, allowing healing by secondary intention with early mobilization and physiotherapy even with a little bit of exposed bone. Typically the outcome is much more dependent on the outlook of patients and their efforts rather than any surgical treatment. I am not aware that any dressing is definitely better than another. If there is good length but loss of much of the pulp, we perform a local flap or even a partial toe transfer for loss of the thumb pulp. Our patients are generally accepting of some shortening so we rarely perform a free toe transfer except in the thumb. It would be wonderful to see a really good trial showing what is best. Currently this is a field dominated by biased opinions. I am sure mine is also biased.

Jin Bo Tang

My approach has evolved over the past 25 years. In my early practice, complex methods were the choice; about 10 years ago, a reverse homodigital pedicled flap or a propeller flap was my main choice. In more recent years, I always explain to the patients 2 ways to treat tip defects: 1 is nonoperative—the tissue regenerate even with distal bone loss, but it may take more than 1 month or 1.5 months; and the other is flap coverage, which is quicker to heal. I almost always use a local advancement flap, such as a Moberg flap, for thumb tip or pulp and volar or bilateral V-Y flap for fingertip or pulp, if the patient prefers a shorter healing time. In recent years I rarely use reverse homodigital pedicled flap and seldom use pedicled thenar flap. I have not used a cross-finger flap for many years, because other options are better than a cross-finger flap. I avoid a method in which donor site is a finger and needs skin graft to cover with poor cosmetics; a cross-finger flap causes such problems, as does a reverse homodigital pedicled flap. It seems to be an unwise decision to have scar in another site on the injured finger or another finger for the sake of repairing a fingertip. For a larger wound, I perform a V-Y flap (volar or bilateral), advancing the V part, leaving 2 mm to 3 mm space with around the V with loose skin suture, to allow skin regeneration. This combines a flap transfer and skin regeneration to cover a defect larger than the flap. The sacrifice is limited! For a larger defect extending over the distal joint or 2 joints, a kite flap is used for thumb or a free vascularized flap from the wrist or forearm for the thumb or finger.

I have found many Asian surgeons have not fully realized the capability of the fingertip to regenerate after injury, and nonsurgical occlusive dressings work well. I also urge colleagues to use a local flap in larger-sized defects, to avoid investing time in complex flaps.

DISTAL DIGITAL TIP REPLANTATION

Question: Distal digital tip replantation (here defined as replantation distal to the midlevel of the distal phalanx) has been reported by several Japanese surgeons; this is also common in quite a few other Asian countries. It is known to many surgeons, however, that the replanted tip often does not have good sensation. Instead, a sensate flap or tip regeneration may lead to better sensory recovery. Views seem different among Asian and European surgeons. Please comment on whether replantation at this level is popular in your practice. Is that true that European surgeons are more inclined not to replant a tip amputation, at least not regularly attempting to replant the very distal tip?

Shohei Omokawa

Although distal finger replantation (Tamai zones 1 and 2) provides excellent cosmetic outcomes by maintaining digital length and nail, the replantation needs special microsurgical techniques and sutures (sometimes 12-0 suture materials). Replantation at this level is not popular in Japan but some enthusiastic surgeons perform this difficult surgery.

I consider that the indications for distal finger replantation are clean-cut or local crush amputation in young and highly motivated patients, especially women, even in elderly patients.

Crush or avulsion amputation may have poor sensory recovery after replantation, because neurorrhaphy and venous anastomosis are difficult or impossible to achieve. I consider that a graft on flap procedure may have better clinical outcomes than replantation surgery.[7]

Thomas Giesen

It is true that in Europe the tendency is to use a sensate flap primarily because of the decreasing funding. Nevertheless, in our practice we actually always look under the microscope to see if the vessels are viable for replantation.

Michel Ernest H. Boeckstyns

I do not consider replantation in these cases but treat as described previously for fingertip soft tissue defects. In small children up to 6 years old, I perform a nonvascularized replantation.

Shian Chao Tay

Distal digital tip replantation is also performed in Singapore with either bleeding or dermal pocketing to manage venous congestion. Another alternative to distal digital replantation is full-thickness perionychial grafting in combination with a local flap.[7] I use this technique with the cross-finger flap and reserve it only for fingertip amputations. The procedure is simple and reliable and patients can be discharged the next day. This technique is not suitable for the thumb due to the increased size of the graft.

Grey Giddins

We rarely replant a fingertip in adults but consider it in children, especially for thumb injuries. In adults I think there is little if any evidence that the attached fingertip recovers in function. Rather it simply acts as a dressing, so we typically treat with a dressing and early therapy, as noted previously.

NO PERIPHERAL TENDON REPAIR

Question: Peripheral sutures of the flexor tendon during primary repair may not be very important if a strong core suture repair is used. I know Dr Giesen does not use peripheral sutures when a 6-strand core repair is used has achieved good outcomes. I remember in the Federation of European Societies for Surgery of the Hand meeting of 2016, pictures in Dr Giesen's presentation showed the contact site diameter of 2 cut stumps was approximately (or more than) 150% that of a normal tendon after completion of the core suture. What is the acceptable bulkiness of the repair site after completion of core sutures that does not hinder active tendon motion? I know hand surgeons in Singapore often use Lim-Tsai repair; is it possible to place all the 6 repair strands in the volar half of the tendons as described?

Thomas Giesen

We know from the published literature that even if the tendon diameter at the repair site is almost equal to the normal tendon, the diameter is approximately 150% at 1 week after surgery, even with a circumferential suture.[8] This observation led us to focus more on the tendon sheath than on the technique itself and to believe that tendon sheath management might be more important than the suturing technique per se. With the core technique we are currently using, it is possible to distribute dorsal/volar 6 strands of the core suture, such that most of the strands are dorsally, and the tendon is realigned without the need of a circumferential suture. The 6 strands seems to provide enough strength that allows immediate digital active mobilization.

Shian Chao Tay

In a recent study of ours, 85% of lacerated flexor tendons were repaired with Lim-Tsai type. It is not necessary to confine the core sutures to the volar half of the repaired tendon.

Jin Bo Tang

I find that peripheral sutures are much less important when a strong core suture is used. I always added peripheral sutures in the past, however, when I used a strong core suture.[9–17] The peripheral sutures that I use now are usually not as standard as we read in textbooks. I put a few running stitches to make the volar gliding surface smoother. Dorsally I do not add peripheral sutures if it is too difficult to turn the tendon. Because I always maintain tension across the core suture, the tendon junction site is a little bulky. I always keep such bulkiness to less than 20% to 30% of the tendon diameter and add a few stitches of peripheral sutures to smoothen the junction.

BONY MALLET FINGERS

Question: There is a recent report in the *Journal of Hand Surgery* (American volume) from Korean surgeons[18] on outcomes of 2 treatments for bony mallet fingers with one-third or more articular surface involvement. They concluded that the clinical outcomes do not significantly differ between extension block pinning and nonsurgical management for mallet fractures involving more than one-third of the articular surface, when the cases do not have a "high degree" of distal interphalangeal (DIP) joint subluxation. I found "high-degree" hard to define. I would like to know the comments from Dr Giddins: what is your guideline? I also would like to know the treatment options and indications of Dr Omokawa (and Japanese colleagues), because the extension block pinning was developed by Japanese colleagues. Would this article change your practice? I appreciate comments on the length of conservative treatment and how to balance fracture healing versus prevention of DIP joint stiffness?

Grey Giddins

The key seems to be subluxation of the main fracture fragment of the distal phalanx. If the main body of the distal phalanx does not sublux, then the outcome is typically very good and there is no evidence that the outcomes from surgery are any better. Therefore, the only sensible aim for surgery seems to reduce and hold the main distal phalanx fracture fragment. That can be done reliably with a single Kirschner (K) wire. There is no evidence that more complicated surgery reliably improves the outcome.

Hyperextension stressing of the distal phalanx, that is, pushing the tip of the finger into extension, seems to predict subluxation of the main distal fracture fragment more than 1 mm to 2 mm reasonably and reliably. Therefore, I test all bony mallet fractures greater than one-third with a hyperextension stress test.[19] If the distal phalanx pivots subluxation is likely. I splint them in slight flexion if not subluxed and watch carefully for 3 weeks. If the fragment is subluxed initially or subsequently, I reduce and fix with an oblique K wire under local anesthesia. I remove the wire in clinic after 5 weeks.

A majority only need splintage. I now splint for 4 weeks to 5 weeks but no more. I suspect that only 3 weeks to 4 weeks is necessary. This is a metaphyseal fracture in the hand so it should heal very quickly and be stable by 4 weeks from injury. I do not think these fractures need splintage for 6 weeks (this is now my practice but unproven); I continue to splint tendinous mallet injuries for at least 6 weeks.

Shohei Omokawa

For a mallet fracture with a large fracture fragment and DIP joint subluxation, I usually use percutaneous extension block and temporary DIP joint fixation (Ishiguro method)[20] using K wires. Although recent hook plates may provide stable fracture fixation,[21] the plating is a less cost effective and less minimally invasive procedure than the percutaneous methods and may have benefit only for patients who hope to avoid pin-site wound problems. Conservative treatment of bony mallet fracture is selected for cases of acceptable joint congruity and no joint subluxation. I believe unstable intra-articular joint fracture should be treated surgically even if it happens in the DIP joint.

Michel Ernest H. Boeckstyns

I am not sure the article by Yoon and colleagues[18] will change my algorithm. My treatment of bony mallet fingers consists of the following:

1. Reducing the extension lag and attempting to reduce subluxation and displacement by close manipulation and applying a palmar splint.
2. If radiographs show minimal displacement or subluxation (this is subjective and hard to define), I continue nonsurgical treatment for 4 weeks to 6 weeks with weekly radiographs at 1 week, 2 weeks, and 4 weeks.
3. If the fragment is more than one-third of the articular surface and there is significant displacement or subluxation after attempting reduction, I go for extension block pinning and protect with a palmar splint for 4 weeks.

Shian Chao Tay

Conservative treatment with a mallet finger splint for 6 weeks is reserved for cases of a fracture too small to be controlled by implants or larger fractures that are in acceptable position and without joint subluxation. For those patients needing surgery, either a hook plate or extension block pinning is used in Singapore, depending on surgeon preference. My preference is hook plate fixation fixation by a K wire through the DIP joint, which I pull out 4 weeks to 6 weeks later; the indications are a large displaced fracture with DIP joint subluxation and significant extensor lag. Indications for surgery are controversial in patients with sizable mallet fractures associated with displacement and/or joint subluxation but without DIP joint extensor lag. My current indications are to offer surgery for displacement more than 2 mm or presence of any joint subluxation.

A small risk of nail deformity with the use of a hook plate exists, which can be minimized by placing the plate under the periosteum of the distal phalanx. Nail deformity may resolve after plate removal when the fracture has healed.

Jin Bo Tang

The literature may give guidance for selection of different methods.[22–24] The displacement of fracture fragment for which surgical block pinning is necessary has not been well defined. I usually consider fracture with approximately one-third or greater joint involvement with seeable radiologic displacement (subluxation) for dorsal blocking pinning. I believe this is a safer way, so I do not need to worry the fragment will displace further later on. Currently, I do not plan to change after reading the recent reports. DIP joint stiffness is common after either conservative or surgical treatment of tendinous mallet finger, which I think needs at least 6 weeks' full-time splinting and splinting for most of the time in a day in the subsequent 2 weeks.

ARTHROSCOPY IN THE PATIENTS WITH DISTAL RADIUS FRACTURE

Question: Not all hand surgeons are familiar with arthroscopic techniques, but a certain (low) percentage of the patients with distal radial fractures have appreciable carpal ligament or triangular fibrocartilage complex (TFCC) tears. I would like to know from Dr Omokawa what your indications are for using an arthroscopy when you treat the distal radius fracture operatively. Do you repair the TFCC injury at the same time of fracture reduction and internal fixation? What is the rate of positive and appreciable ligament tears you can detect when you surgically treat the distal radius fracture? What are the views of Drs Tay, Boeckstyns, and Giddins, even if some of you may not perform arthroscopy?

Shohei Omokawa

I use wrist arthroscopy routinely when surgical treatment is selected for intra-articular distal radius fractures. The purpose of arthroscopy is to inspect any intra-articular gaps and steps in the articular surface of the distal radius as well as to examine ligament tears and cartilage damage. The magnitude of intra-articular displacement can be directly observed with arthroscopy; this displacement is usually minimal after adequate open reduction of the metaphyseal displacement and percutaneous fixation of distal fracture fragments by interfragmentary K wires under fluoroscopic control.

My colleagues and I have prospectively studied 163 consecutive patients with unstable distal radius fractures treated with volar locking plating; among these patients, complete radioulnar ligament tears of the distal radioulnar joint (DRUJ) instability were present in 11 (7%) of the 163 fractures, which were all confirmed through an open approach and repaired at the same time as fracture fixation.[25] Our other data showed that a traumatic TFCC tear was seen in 159 wrists (45%), and a foveal tear with instability of the ulnar head was repaired primarily in 4 wrists (1.4%). A scapholunate (SL) interosseous ligament injury was seen in 88 wrists (32%). Of these, a complete tear was seen only in 5 (2%) wrists, 4 of which were repaired at the time of surgical treatment of distal radius fractures.

Wrist arthroscopy reveals useful information in patients with intra-articular distal radius fractures. Robust evidence is lacking to date, however, regarding the benefit to the final outcomes of the patients, which further studies need to clarify.

Shian Chao Tay

I reserve arthroscopically assisted fixation of distal radius fractures for isolated die punch fractures with more than 2-mm step-off or persistent remarkable articular incongruity of more than 2 mm after open reduction and internal fixation. Otherwise, I do not use an arthroscope during distal radius fixations. I routinely check DRUJ stability during anesthesia, however, by performing a DRUJ displacement test after fixation of the distal radius fracture, with the forearm in neutral. If there is a remarkably increased displacement compared with the normal side, or if there is loss of volar or dorsal endpoints, the DRUJ is deemed unstable. If the DRUJ is reduced, I put the patient on a Muenster splint in neutral forearm position for 6 weeks. I perform an open TFCC repair and pinning through the DRUJ in its reduced position with the forearm in neutral when there is persistent DRUJ subluxation.

Michel Ernest H. Boeckstyns

In cases of extra-articular fractures, I do not perform arthroscopy, unless radiographs suggest an SL ligament tear or DRUJ subluxation. When treating intraarticular fractures, I increasingly use arthroscopy to assist and assess reduction. If I find a dissociative SL lesion or a peripheral TFCC avulsion, I repair it. For small tears, I may apply a splint for 6 weeks. I have no precise figure concerning the occurrence of appreciable ligament lesions but perform ligament repair in fewer than 10% of intra-articular fractures.

Grey Giddins

I rarely do this. There is no evidence that it improves outcomes. TFCC injuries are common; leaving them does not seem to lead to a poor outcome. By using a customized jig, we have recently shown that all distal radius fractures have a persistent DRUJ injury with some measurable instability but it rarely causes problems. Together these imply we are not necessarily looking at the material problem when we assess these injuries. In the main, convex joint, surfaces are reasonably forgiving; hence, some distal radius malalignment is well tolerated by most patients. To make progress, a randomized controlled trial of arthroscopic and nonarthroscopic assisted fracture fixation is needed to answer this question. Anything less will almost certainly add nothing to current knowledge.

Jin Bo Tang

In my department, 4 surgical teams are led by 5 senior surgeons. The use of arthroscopy in distal radius fractures depends on whether the senior surgeons like arthroscopy. One team uses arthroscopy for all surgically treated cases of intra-articular distal radius fractures; more than 300 patients have had arthroscopically assisted reduction and assessment of ligament conditions. They have found this approach is helpful to ascertain that the step-off resolves adequately after reduction and to reduce die punch fractures. Few (less than 5% of) patients, however, were found to have ligamentous disruption that needed surgical repair. These surgeons are continuing with this approach, but I have advised them to consider not performing arthroscopy in all these surgical cases, rather, to do it more selectively according to the severity of the intra-articular fractures. The surgeons in the other 2 teams do not use arthroscopy at all. They consider that few patients have ligament injuries that require immediate attention; for those few patients who need repair, later treatment is probably enough. My thought is that arthroscopy is useful for those with severely displaced intra-articular fractures. Similar to isolated carpal ligament injuries,[26–30] partial tear or elongation of ligaments with the fracture are common under the scope, but they do not need surgical repair; whether immediate repair of the disrupted ligaments is necessary is unclear.

The expertise of surgeons who perform arthroscopy greatly affects repair outcomes. I recommend the outcomes be reported together with the level of the expertise of surgeons who perform arthroscopic repairs, similar to those recent reports of hand surgery.[31–37]

QUESTIONABLE CLINICAL DIAGNOSIS

Question: In hand surgery, there are some diagnoses that not all hand surgeons agree on or believe really exist. These conditions may include thoracic outlet syndrome, CRPS, radial tunnel syndrome, pronator syndrome, and radial tunnel syndrome. Please indicate which one or several that you have never seen in your practice or do not believe exist. Please also comment on those others that you have encountered and whether you have ever made the diagnosis. I think these diseases and their diagnosis are still subject to a lot of disagreement.

Michel Ernest H. Boeckstyns

I believe all these conditions exist but they are difficult to define, diagnose, and treat. Diagnosis is mainly based on clinical judgment; this implies a certain degree of subjective evaluation. Neurophysiology, CT, MRI, and ultrasonography do not have a high sensitivity or specificity, thus have no useful predictive value on the outcome of treatment. To the list, I add quadrilateral space

syndrome, compression of the suprascapular nerve, double crush syndrome, and even multiple crush syndrome. Nevertheless, I am convinced that they exist and have encountered them all. The most difficult cases are those of symptomatology dominated by pain or with no or little motor deficit. It is crucial try to differentiate between CRPS and nerve compression. I have operated on several unusual compression syndromes with a rate of success of no more than 50%.

Grey Giddins

I believe they all exist. Apart from CRPS, most are rare and some rarer than others. The problem is a lack of reliable diagnostic tools. When a diagnosis is clearly shown, such as vascular studies proving thoracic outlet syndrome, then surgery is appropriate. For most of these conditions, I recommend a second opinion and waiting a good long time before operating. I suspect many patients will recover and are only assisted by the placebo effect of surgery (see Ian Harris's book, *Surgery the Ultimate Placebo*). Interesting questions are, How many surgeons would have operations on themselves for these conditions and under what criteria? and How long would they wait?

CRPS is complex. CRPS II is clear. CRPS I is more challenging. I suspect that many (not all) cases of CRPS are due to underlying pathology be it a nerve injury or perhaps joint mal-alignment that may be amenable to further treatment. Often it is difficult to differentiate true CRPS from an overreaction to injury/surgery. The key for me is early diagnosis and treatment. The vast majority can be resolved; once well established, CRPS I can be extremely difficult to treat.

Shohei Omokawa

I have experienced several cases with each of these peripheral nerve–related syndromes. Despite theses rare occasions, I consider that each syndrome does exist. The diagnostic criteria, however, have not yet been established. Thus, a prospective multicenter cohort study is needed to reach a consensus on this issue.

Thomas Giesen

I have experienced and diagnosed all of the diagnoses listed previously. Cases of thoracic outlet syndrome referred by our vascular surgeons because of a vascular problem typically have an extra rib.

Shian Chao Tay

The conditions listed are indeed rare. In my outpatient registry of more than 23,000 patient entries since 2009, I have only diagnosed 2 patients with radial tunnel and 2 patients with pronator syndrome. I also have a few patients with CRPS and my department has operated on a few cases of thoracic outlet syndrome over the years.

By the way, it has been believed that ulnostyloid impingement is rare. In my experience, it is a common diagnosis. An audit of my wrist registry showed that nearly one-quarter of patients with wrist pain have ulnostyloid impingement. The provocative test is the Ruby test, that is, tenderness at the tip of the ulnar styloid and/or the dorsal triquetrum.[38] Radiographs rarely show abnormalities. This is largely a clinical diagnosis based on the Ruby test and provoked pain in the correct site. Most patients improve with conservative management with 6 weeks of a neutral wrist splint; avoidance of wrist dorsiflexion, supination, ulnar deviation, and axial loading and its combinations; and topical anti-inflammatory medications.

REFERENCES

1. Mitsunaga N, Mihara M, Koshima I, et al. Digital artery perforator (DAP) flaps: modifications for fingertip and finger stump reconstruction. J Plast Reconstr Aesthet Surg 2010;63:1312–7.

2. Chen C, Tang P, Zhang X. The dorsal homodigital island flap based on the dorsal branch of the digital artery: a review of 166 cases. Plast Reconstr Surg 2014;133:519e–29e.

3. Lim GJ, Yam AK, Lee JY, et al. The spiral flap for fingertip resurfacing: short-term and long-term results. J Hand Surg Am 2008;33:340–7.

4. Adani R, Busa R, Castagnetti C, et al. Homodigital neurovascular island flaps with "direct flow" vascularization. Ann Plast Surg 1997;38:36–40.

5. Teoh LC, Tay SC, Yong FC, et al. Heterodigital arterialized flaps for large finger wounds: results and indications. Plast Reconstr Surg 2003;111:1905–13.

6. Tay SC, Teoh LC, Tan SH, et al. Extending the reach of the heterodigital arterialized flap by vein division and repair. Plast Reconstr Surg 2004;114:1450–6.

7. Netscher DT, Meade RA. Reconstruction of fingertip amputations with full-thickness perionychial grafts from the retained part and local flaps. Plast Reconstr Surg 1999;104:1705–12.

8. Puippe GD, Lindenblatt N, Gnannt R, et al. Morphologic and dynamic morphological assessment of deep flexor tendon healing in zone II by high-frequency ultrasound: preliminary experience. AJR Am J Roentgenol 2011;197:W1110–7.

9. Tang JB, Amadio PC, Boyer MI, et al. Current practice of primary flexor tendon repair: a global view. Hand Clin 2013;29:179–89.

10. Tang JB. Indications, methods, postoperative motion and outcome evaluation of primary flexor tendon repairs in Zone 2. J Hand Surg Eur Vol 2007;32:118–29.

11. Tang JB, Shi D, Gu YQ, et al. Double and multiple looped suture tendon repair. J Hand Surg Br 1994;19:699–703.

12. Tang JB. Outcomes and evaluation of flexor tendon repair. Hand Clin 2013;29:251–9.

13. Zhou X, Li XR, Qing J, et al. Outcomes of the 6-strand M-Tang repair for zone 2 primary flexor tendon repair in 54 fingers. J Hand Surg Eur Vol 2017;42:462–8.

14. Tang JB. Clinical outcomes associated with flexor tendon repair. Hand Clin 2005;21:199–210.

15. Moriya K, Yoshizu T, Tsubokawa N, et al. Outcomes of release of the entire A4 pulley after flexor tendon repairs in zone 2A followed by early active mobilization. J Hand Surg Eur Vol 2016;41:400–5.

16. Moriya K, Yoshizu T, Maki Y, et al. Clinical outcomes of early active mobilization following flexor tendon repair using the six-strand technique: short- and long-term evaluations. J Hand Surg Eur Vol 2015;40:250–8.

17. Edsfeldt S, Rempel D, Kursa K, et al. In vivo flexor tendon forces generated during different rehabilitation exercises. J Hand Surg Eur Vol 2015;40:705–10.

18. Yoon JO, Baek H, Kim JK. The outcomes of extension block pinning and nonsurgical management for mallet fracture. J Hand Surg Am 2017;42(5):387.e1–7.

19. Giddins GE. Bony mallet finger injuries: assessment of stability with extension stress testing. J Hand Surg Eur Vol 2016;41:696–700.

20. Pegoli L, Toh S, Arai K, et al. The Ishiguro extension block technique for the treatment of mallet finger fracture: indications and clinical results. J Hand Surg Br 2003;28:15–7.

21. Toker S, Türkmen F, Pekince O, et al. Extension block pinning versus hook plate fixation for treatment of mallet fractures. J Hand Surg Am 2015;40:1591–6.

22. Elzinga KE, Chung KC. Finger Injuries in football and rugby. Hand Clin 2017;33:149–60.

23. Acar MA, Güzel Y, Güleç A, et al. Clinical comparison of hook plate fixation versus extension block pinning for bony mallet finger: a retrospective comparison study. J Hand Surg Eur Vol 2015;40:832–9.

24. Wada T, Oda T. Mallet fingers with bone avulsion and DIP joint subluxation. J Hand Surg Eur Vol 2015;40:8–15.

25. Fujitani R, Omokawa S, Akahane M, et al. Predictors of distal radioulnar joint instability in distal radius fractures. J Hand Surg Am 2011;36:1919–25.

26. Lindau TR. The role of arthroscopy in carpal instability. J Hand Surg Eur Vol 2016;41:35–47.

27. Koehler SM, Guerra SM, Kim JM, et al. Outcome of arthroscopic reduction association of the scapholunate joint. J Hand Surg Eur Vol 2016;41:48–55.

28. van de Grift TC, Ritt MJ. Management of lunotrique-tral instability: a review of the literature. J Hand Surg Eur Vol 2016;41:72–85.

29. Tosti R, Shin E. Wrist arthroscopy for athletic injuries. Hand Clin 2017;33:107–17.

30. Desai MJ, Kamal RN, Richard MJ. Management of intercarpal ligament injuries associated with distal radius fractures. Hand Clin 2015;31:409–16.

31. Tang JB, Giddins G. Why and how to report surgeons' levels of expertise. J Hand Surg Eur Vol 2016;41:365–6.

32. Tang JB. Re: levels of experience of surgeons in clinical studies. J Hand Surg Eur Vol 2009;34:137–8.

33. Storey PA, Goddard M, Clegg C, et al. Pyrocarbon proximal interphalangeal joint arthroplasty: a medium to long term follow-up of a single surgeon series. J Hand Surg Eur Vol 2015;40:952–6.

34. Mattila S, Waris E. Unfavourable short-term outcomes of a poly-L/D-lactide scaffold for thumb trapeziometacarpal arthroplasty. J Hand Surg Eur Vol 2016;41:328–34.

35. Frueh FS, Kunz VS, Gravestock IJ. Primary flexor tendon repair in zones 1 and 2: early passive mobilization versus controlled active motion. J Hand Surg Am 2014;39:1344–50.

36. Moriya K, Yoshizu T, Tsubokawa N, et al. Clinical results of releasing the entire A2 pulley after flexor tendon repair in zone 2C. J Hand Surg Eur Vol 2016;41:822–8.

37. Moriya K, Yoshizu T, Tsubokawa N, et al. Outcomes of flexor tendon repairs in zone 2 subzones with early active mobilization. J Hand Surg Eur Vol 2017. http://dx.doi.org/10.1177/1753193417715213.

38. Topper SM, Wood MB, Ruby LK. Ulnar styloid impaction syndrome. J Hand Surg Am 1997;22:699–704.

Moving?

Make sure your subscription moves with you!

To notify us of your new address, find your **Clinics Account Number** (located on your mailing label above your name), and contact customer service at:

Email: journalscustomerservice-usa@elsevier.com

800-654-2452 (subscribers in the U.S. & Canada)
314-447-8871 (subscribers outside of the U.S. & Canada)

Fax number: 314-447-8029

Elsevier Health Sciences Division
Subscription Customer Service
3251 Riverport Lane
Maryland Heights, MO 63043

*To ensure uninterrupted delivery of your subscription, please notify us at least 4 weeks in advance of move.

ELSEVIER